ABORIGINAL SECRETS
OF AWAKENING

"Get comfortable and start reading. You'll be transported into a dynamic world that gives insight, value, and hope for a future you can help design."

DONNA SEEBO, HOST OF *THE DONNA SEEBO SHOW*

"In this book, Robbie's surrender to the transformative power of love shines a bright beacon on our own quest for wholeness."

JIM MACARTNEY, AUTHOR OF *CRISIS TO CREATION*

"*Aboriginal Secrets of Awakening* is a profound journey into the ancient Aboriginal healings and the power of the human spirit and mind in the ability to heal as choice not chance. A must-read for anyone challenged with a chronic illness."

SONIA TREJO, HEALTH AND WELLNESS COACH AND FOUNDER OF THE ALCHEMY OF HOPE AND HEALING

"If you have ever wondered 'Why do bad things happen to good people?' then *Aboriginal Secrets of Awakening* will help you to understand how all exists for a higher good, which is the basis of All that is."

SUSAN E. KOLB, M.D., F.A.C.S., HOST OF *TEMPLE OF HEALTH RADIO SHOW*

"From the first page, Robbie draws you so deeply into experiencing her life that by the final page you feel a connection with her husband so palpable you can feel his presence. This book is a must-read for spiritual seekers, those curious about alternative healing, and anyone who savors romance."

LEAH GRANT, INTUITIVE, SPEAKER, AUTHOR, AND CREATOR OF ECSTATIC MEDITATION

"Gleaned from the timelessness of ancient wisdom, *Aboriginal Secrets of Awakening* holds the key to understanding self-healing on a mind, body, and spirit level."

LINDA MACKENZIE, HOST OF
GM-HEALTHYLIFE.NET RADIO NETWORK

"This book will take readers on a journey as they learn to live their passions and free themselves from their health and life challenges and move from sickness to wellness."

STEPHANIE E. TIPPIE, RRT,
COHOST OF AGING YOUNGER RADIO

"A moving memoir of an extraordinary journey, courageous in its intimacy, this is a story of miraculous healing and an adventure into the world of spirit that demonstrates the challenges and the rewards of the sacred quest for wholeness in mind, body, and spirit."

MARILYN MCGUIRE, FOUNDER OF NAUTILUS BOOK AWARDS

"Brilliantly reveals the secrets of the spiritual world—how to live an illuminated life. Well done!"

"SONJAN" DAVID CHRISTOPHER MCCOMBS,
COAUTHOR OF *APPRENTICESHIP OF THE SOUL*

"*Aboriginal Secrets of Awakening* is beautifully written. An inspiring memoir that will move you deeply."

KAREN R. PERKINS, D.B.A., CPM,
PERSONAL GROWTH CONSULTANT AND TRAINER

"Beautifully told, *Aboriginal Secrets of Awakening* ranks up there with the most compelling books to cherish."

STARFEATHER MARCY, SPIRITUAL TEACHER, HEALER,
ARTIST, AND MEDICINE WOMAN

"*Aboriginal Secrets of Awakening* not only makes me grateful for my own health and for those around me but also captivates and inspires further hope beyond the traditional medicine approach."

JEN BLAU, CPT, WELLNESS COACH

ABORIGINAL SECRETS
OF AWAKENING

A JOURNEY OF HEALING
AND SPIRITUALITY WITH A
REMOTE AUSTRALIAN TRIBE

ROBBIE HOLZ
WITH CHRISTIANN HOWARD

Bear & Company
Rochester, Vermont • Toronto, Canada

Bear & Company
One Park Street
Rochester, Vermont 05767
www.BearandCompanyBooks.com

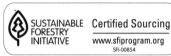

Text stock is SFI certified

Bear & Company is a division of Inner Traditions International

Library of Congress Cataloging-in-Publication Data
Holz, Robbie.
    Aboriginal secrets of awakening : a journey of healing and spirituality with a
remote Australian tribe / Robbie Holz.
        p. cm.
    Summary: "One woman's story of healing through Aboriginal principles and
awakening to her own healing powers" — Provided by publisher.
    ISBN 978-1-59143-219-7 (pbk.) — ISBN 978-1-59143-220-3 (e-book)
                                                                    2014042347

Printed and bound in the United States by Lake Book Manufacturing, Inc.
The text stock is SFI certified. The Sustainable Forestry Initiative® program
promotes sustainable forest management.

10 9 8 7 6 5 4 3 2 1

Text design and layout by Virginia Scott Bowman
This book was typeset in Garamond Premier Pro and ITC Legacy Sans Std with
Gill Sans MT Pro used as the display typeface

To send correspondence to the author of this book, mail a first-class letter to the
author c/o Inner Traditions • Bear & Company, One Park Street, Rochester, VT
05767, and we will forward the communication, or contact the author directly at
www.holzwellness.com.

*This book is dedicated to Gary, Mother Mary,
the remote Australian Aborigines, and the rest
of my spirit team (you know who you are).
I love you.*

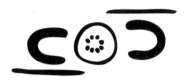

As with any memoir, the stories in this book are true.

With the exception of Gary and myself, the names, physical descriptions, and in some cases the occupations, of the persons in this book have been changed to protect the privacy of the individuals involved.

Also, to protect the privacy of individuals in the small towns where we lived and practiced, Archer, Benton, Keyserville, and Richards are fictitious names for towns in Washington state. Eleanor is a fictitious name for a town in Canada. However, their settings and attributes are real.

The name Jaripuyjangu, which is used for the name of the Aboriginal tribe that hosted our group of women for ceremony, is also fictional. To protect the privacy of the individuals involved, I have combined selected syllables from the names of several Aboriginal tribes to create a fictional Aboriginal tribal name. However, the tribe is real, as are all the experiences in Australia that I describe.

The testimonials and "thank you" cards that were received from grateful patients and included in this book are real. They are reprinted here in their own words with the patients' permission. Only the names and initials have been changed to protect their privacy.

CONTENTS

	Acknowledgments	xi
	Prologue: Journeys and Windows	xiii
1	Gunner	1
2	The Perfect Setup	6
3	An Arm Full of Scars	13
4	One Crash Is Not Enough	17
5	Good-Bye Memory	23
6	A Visit with Grandpa Homer	28
7	Herbs and Potions After All	34
8	Flying Down the Path	39
9	"I Am Not a Teacher!"	46
10	Regarding Soul Mates	51
11	A Quiet Man	57
12	A Job Offer	61
13	Ann	66
14	A Suddenness of Love	71

15	Gary's Trip to Australia	75
16	Yes, a Healer	80
17	Many Lives	84
18	Miracle upon Miracle	89
19	Ditto	94
20	A Honeymoon	96
21	Healing of a Skeptic	100
22	The Power of a Focused Mind	103
23	Why Is the Great Healer in a Wheelchair?	108
24	A Soul's Purpose	113
25	The Quest to Walk	121
26	Four Out of Five Ain't Bad	124
27	Ray	127
28	The Root of an Illness	131
29	A Long and Lovely Song	136
30	Yeah? Well, Read This!	139
31	Lynn Arrives	141
32	Remote Healing	146
33	Checker Helping	152
34	Spirit Guides	156
35	Guiding Meditation	160
36	Starting before the Problem Arises	164
37	The Dark Side of Caregiving	168
38	A Lesson in Gratitude	172

39	Waiting	180
40	The Gathering at the Crossing	184
41	The Last Precious Gifts	189
42	Finally Dancing	192
43	Still a Team	195
44	A Second Wooing	198
45	Accepting Love	202
46	My Checker-Helping Mind	207
47	An Apartment	211
48	Preparing for Australia	218
49	Light for the Lightworkers	222
50	Camping	229
51	Sacred Fires	237
52	A Mother's Love	245
53	Thunderstorms	248
54	A Blessing	253
55	Rebirth from the Womb of Uluru	256
56	The Right Alignment	259
57	Home Is Where . . .	265
58	Paris	269
	Continuing the Journey	272

ACKNOWLEDGMENTS

This book exists because of the dedication, skills, and support of many people.

I am deeply grateful to my dear friend Christiann Howard for using her extraordinary talents and tireless devotion toward creating this book.

I wish to express particular appreciation to Ron and Barbara Carstens.

For their immeasurable contributions to this book, I am extremely grateful to the following: Helen Howard, Kim Votry, Janette Turner, Charles Noble, Billy Heath, Laurie Holderman, Raven Neumann, Danielle Gibbons, Olga Teisseyre, and Kathy Logan.

I extend heartfelt gratitude and love to all of you.

JOURNEYS AND WINDOWS

One summer when I was a child, my family took a car trip across the Painted Desert to the Grand Canyon, and we kids fought constantly over the window seats. There were five of us kids—four in the backseat because there were no seat belts back then—and after every rest stop, getting us back into the car was a tussle.

"You get in first, Ann. It's my turn to be by the window."

"It is not."

"You were by it before lunch!"

"And you were by it all morning before Albuquerque."

"Mo-oooom! It's my turn."

Adult intervention: "Robbie. Get in the car."

"But—"

Adult determination: "I don't want to hear it. Get in the car!"

You get the idea. We used to fight for the window seats. The thing is, I have no idea why.

I didn't actually enjoy looking out the window. The desert stretched away on all sides in folded layers of fantastically colored rock—rust red, smoky gray, and ochre yellow—but I didn't see the

beauty. I only saw a barren desert. I just wanted to sleep through it.
Wake me up when we get there, okay?
All across the Painted Desert, eating spam sandwiches in the heat—
that's what I remember. Not the spectacular Grand Canyon.
Wake me up when we get there.
Then life proceeded. And somewhere along the line—after I grew
up, and managed to achieve what I had been striving so hard to achieve,
and then found that my achievements didn't bring me the meaning and
joy I had hoped for—I began to wake up to the trip.

I woke up to a whole universe behind the universe. I woke up to the
pattern and the presence of the Divine behind all of creation, behind
everything—even behind me! And that's when I discovered that a desert isn't really a desert at all.

My husband, Gary Holz, made his own trip into the desert. He
journeyed to the Australian Outback in 1994 to stay with a remote
Aboriginal tribe. He was seeking a cure for his progressive multiple
sclerosis (MS). In Australia, he experienced a miraculous improvement
in his physical condition. Feeling returned to parts of his body that had
been numb for seven years. He had been bound to a wheelchair for two
years and, on the trip home, he clumsily walked down the airplane aisle.
The first book we wrote together, *Secrets of Aboriginal Healing,* is the
story of that trip.

When he returned, he never became completely free of the wheelchair, and eventually (more than a decade after the doctors said he
would) he left his physical form. But that is only a tiny fraction of his
truth. After Gary returned from the Outback, he became a conduit
for miraculous healing energy. And hundreds of people benefited from
it—a gift sent from the Australian Aborigines.

Years later, I traveled to the same desert to camp with other members of the same Aboriginal tribe. On my trip, I experienced a miraculous transformation of my own. But my transformation was less about
physical healing and more about self-empowerment.

This is the story of those several journeys: Gary's journey through life after he returned from Australia, my life journey before Gary, and both our journeys together. It is the story of how I met Gary, fell in love with him, married him, worked beside him, lost him in his physical form, rediscovered him in his spiritual form, and continued on, constantly made aware of his love and the love of the rest of my personal spiritual team.

Looking back, I can see it was an inward journey. A journey to awareness. And I had the perfect seat—no need to fight for the window in this case. My love story with Gary? That was definitely a large part of the trip. But it turned out that it was also about my love story with *myself.* Somehow along the way I learned to love myself. And I mean to really love my self, with Divine Love.

How does a person learn to do that? The first thing I did was to roll down the window and start to look for it. Divine Love? Once you start to look—you see it everywhere. And then, after a time of amazement and excitement, a funny thing happens. What you are looking at changes you. One way or another it's not just the window that's open.

It's you.

And the light is streaming in.

You've opened up.

With me, it didn't happen all at once. Sometimes it was like breaking open a melon or an egg—hard and sudden. And sometimes, it was like breathing in a soft breeze until I realized that same breeze was blowing through me as if I were a loosely woven cloth.

Everyone's story is different, and this is mine. Like all memoirs it is a true story. It is *my* truth, my experience.

Though this book's title contains the word *Secrets,* its intent is exactly the opposite. Gary and I, and the Australian Aboriginal communities who charged us with bringing their principles into the world, want to spread the secrets. May these stories inspire you to discover your own secrets of awakening.

1

GUNNER

A single tear traced its way down Kevin's face. He was normally so taciturn, so emotionally controlled, that the sight of it broke my heart. He had one arm around his wife, Kiera. With the other hand he was fondling little Gunner's ear. Gunner was a black and white terrier mix. The way Kiera was nestling the sweet guy in her arms, I could tell he was their baby.

They had just gotten the worst diagnosis a pet owner can get.

These folks have to be exhausted, I thought. They had just returned from Hawaii on a ten-hour flight. I knew they weren't well off, so it must have been a once-in-a-lifetime trip. And here they were in a crisis situation before they could even unpack.

Kevin, Kiera, and I were in an examination room at Dr. Hamilton's veterinary office where I worked as a veterinary assistant. Gunner had been a regular patient of the clinic since puppyhood. Only for the regular shots and exams, though—nothing serious before this.

Earlier on, I was keeping them company while we waited for Dr. Hamilton to fit this emergency in between her already scheduled appointments, and they told me the whole sad story.

Kevin and Kiera had left Gunner in the care of some friends while they went on vacation. As soon as they arrived back in Seattle, Kiera had gone to pick up Gunner at their friends' house. "I missed Gunner so much," she told me brokenly. "The shuttle dropped us home, I set down my bag in the hall, and went right back out the door to go get him."

Right away, she had noticed something was not quite right with Gunner, but she hadn't wanted to make a fuss. Their friends had been doing them a big favor, watching him while they were on this special vacation. She quickly collected Gunner and brought him home for a closer look.

At home it became apparent that something was terribly wrong. Gunner was dragging his hind legs. They just flopped along behind him. He had no control over them at all and he seemed to be in pain. Kevin called the friends who had been watching him.

"Gunner can't move his back legs. Was he like that at your house?"

At first, the family who had been watching Gunner denied knowing anything about it. But Kevin persisted. Eventually, the dad broke down in tears and explained what had happened. They had a developmentally disabled nephew who had visited while they were watching Gunner. Their nephew had trouble controlling his emotions in new situations. They hadn't watched his interaction with the dog closely enough. He had been playing with Gunner and grown frustrated that the little dog wouldn't give him the ball. So the nephew kicked him. Gunner hadn't "been walking right" since, but they were hoping it would take care of itself. They were so sorry.

Later, in the examination room, Dr. Hamilton put the x-rays on the light box. "You can see the breaks here and here. I'm afraid our options are very limited," she said, as she stroked Gunner's head. "With multiple breaks like these, putting him to sleep would be the humane thing to do."

There was a long pause. "No, no," Kiera softly murmured.

"I'm sorry. I wish I could do more. There's no chance he'll ever walk again, and he'll probably always be in pain. I'll leave you for a while to talk about it. Take all the time you need." Dr. Hamilton slipped from the room leaving the couple to their grief . . . and their decision.

Kiera cradled the little guy carefully in her arms. Gunner shivered every so often and a soft whine would escape.

I had been a veterinary assistant to Dr. Hamilton for a year now. She was a marvelous, compassionate veterinarian and a supportive employer. It wasn't her fault she had nothing more to offer. I lingered awkwardly in the examining room. I should leave them to it, give them space. But my heart just wouldn't let me. I was wrestling with my own decision . . .

I had met someone at a party. It was a party given by a friend of mine who had, shall we say . . . unusual abilities. Many of her friends had . . . unusual abilities. This man I had met at the party had traveled to the Outback of Australia and lived with a remote Aboriginal tribe. He had come back from that trip with . . . well . . . miraculous healing abilities. And he worked with animals. I had never personally seen any of his astonishing healings, but I had heard stories.

His name was Dr. Gary Holz.

Should I tell Kiera and Kevin about him? I was unsure. I knew that there were alternatives when traditional medicine had nothing more to offer. I, myself, would not have been alive and working here if that were not true. Why not see if they wanted to give it a try? But I was a veterinarian's assistant. Was it even ethical to suggest an alternative?

While I dithered, Kevin continued to pet Gunner's head with a tear escaping every so often, unnoticed. Neither of them said anything. They both just gazed at Gunner and took turns stroking him. Kiera swallowed painfully. The tears and that swallow decided me.

"I know an alternative healer who might be able to help Gunner."

"Alternative healer?"

"I'm not sure how he does what he does, but I've heard that he's been able to help in situations like this. If you want to give him a try, I'll call him."

They looked at each other. I saw in that look something I would see many times in the years ahead—a faint glimmer of hope where before there had been only dark despair.

Kevin nodded. "Okay. If there's any chance at all . . ."

I called Gary Holz and explained the situation. His response was, "I'll be right there."

Dr. Hamilton was kind enough—and egoless enough—to let Gary come to her office and use her facilities to take a look at Gunner. She greeted him at the door with a handshake and a smile.

If the couple were surprised when Gary rolled into the examining room in a wheelchair, they were too polite to show it. Since I had already met Gary, I wasn't shocked that he was a paraplegic. I felt some admiration as I looked at him sitting there so composed, slim and well-dressed, his hair and beard immaculately trimmed. He seemed to exude a compassion and confidence that filled the space. I felt everyone relax ever so slightly.

I explained about Gunner's broken spine as Gary looked at the x-rays still on the light box. He listened gravely. You got the impression from his clear, observant eyes that he had a staggering intelligence, but he said very little. "Let's see what we can do," he said.

Kiera gently eased Gunner back onto the examination table.

We all watched with hopeful anticipation as Gary rolled his wheelchair alongside Gunner and gently placed his left hand in the middle of Gunner's spine. Gunner became very calm and lay patient and still. No one spoke. To our eyes, nothing more appeared to happen.

After a few minutes, Gary removed his hand and said he thought he could help. He would like to see Gunner again a few more times. We would have to wait and see, but he would do his best.

The tearful couple seemed quite relieved. They offered to pay Gary, but he refused to take their money that day. "I'll be more than happy to help Gunner if I can," he said.

Kiera faithfully brought Gunner to Gary's small clinic several times over the next few weeks. Since I had recommended Gary to Kiera and Kevin, I arranged to go with her. And if the truth be told, I really loved that scrappy little Gunner and I wanted to see what would happen.

Gary's clinic was airy and bright with healthy plants scattered around and impressionist prints on the walls. I realized that the polished parquet floors were to make things easier for Gary's wheelchair. Gary greeted us at the door and ushered us back to his treatment room. Each time we brought Gunner in, Gary would do the same thing. We would place Gunner on the examining table, and Gary would roll alongside in his wheelchair. Then, Gary would place his left hand on the site of the injury for about five minutes, and Gunner would calm down and lie there quietly, breathing slowly.

After the treatment, Gary would put Gunner on the floor saying, "Let's see how he does," and we would all watch to see if Gunner could stand or walk. Ignoring his infirmity, Gunner would explore the office floor, dragging his rear feet behind him.

One day as Gary and I were following Kiera into Gary's treatment room, Gary softly called my name. "Robbie."

"Yes?" I asked, bending down to hear him.

"I want you to watch closely today."

"Okay," I replied, feeling a little thrill of excitement. *Did that mean today would be different?*

Gary rolled his wheelchair to the table and placed his hand on Gunner as usual. When I think of Gary now, I often see him in this characteristic pose: sitting in his wheelchair next to the patient, his head bent, looking slightly down, and with his left hand gently placed upon the injured site. Focused, but peaceful.

To my eyes, the treatment was exactly like the other treatments had been. But this time when Gary placed the little dog on the floor, Gunner pulled his legs under himself, and—while everyone in the room cheered and hugged and cried . . .

Gunner walked.

2

THE PERFECT SETUP

The healing of little Gunner took place in the fall of 2001. I had only recently met Gary and didn't know him well. But I had the confidence to call him to see if he could help Gunner because I knew alternative medical practices could sometimes produce miraculous results. I had already seen someone experience healing through an alternative medical system when all else failed. That someone was me.

My illness began many years before at the time of my son's birth. When I contracted the disease, I didn't know it had happened. It was years before I knew that I had been infected with a disease that would eventually rob me of my vitality, my mobility, my family life, and even my ability to think.

When my son was born in 1985, it was a hard delivery, because his shoulder wasn't in the right position. Thankfully, my medical team and I managed it, but that thirty-six-hour delivery took a lot out of me.

I was lying in my hospital bed feeling totally exhausted and wondering, *How am I ever going to take care of this newborn baby when they send me home? What if I still feel like this? I wonder how long it will take me to get my strength back.*

Then a nurse came to talk with me. "How are you doing?"

"I feel so weak. Will my energy come back soon?"

"That's why I'm here. It's perfectly normal to lose some blood during a birth. We can give you a blood transfusion. It'll perk you up faster."

"Sure!" I croaked.

I was a little distracted at that moment. All I really cared about was the little miracle in my arms. He had to be the sweetest baby ever born. The best day of my life would also be the day I unknowingly opened the door to my greatest nightmare.

I had no idea about the risks of getting someone else's blood—back then they didn't do the blood screening that they do today.

The transfusion I got was tainted with hepatitis C.

In 1985, the disease was not even recognized by the medical community. It's called a "silent killer," because it remains hidden for years as it quietly replicates itself into legions of deadly organisms feeding on many parts of the body at once. Like a Trojan horse, the virus hid in my body—until it confidently and openly declared war seven years later.

When my son turned seven, I was working as a successful court stenographer—clicking through the halls in my red high heels, joking with attorneys and judges, listening to the fascinating cases that came through the courts. I loved it. As a court stenographer I was highly respected. I had passed all the tests for speed and accuracy a person could pass. I had all the initials that you could get for proficiencies in court stenography appearing after my name.

Aaron and I had a good marriage. We were best friends, living the American dream. Aaron had been my high school sweetheart. We had married in a tiny Midwest town on the coldest day of the year. We had moved to the West Coast. We had worked like slaves, and now we were reaping the benefits.

Aaron was an exciting man. He raced cars, motorcycles, snowmobiles, and boats. He flew planes. He was a big, open-hearted man with an infectious enthusiasm for life. Everyone loved him. Aaron and I were both still working full time and investing in other projects in our "spare time." *Let's buy a marina! Why not? We love boats.*

My son had also gotten into racing (yeah, a seven-year-old racing cars on a race track wearing a crash helmet). He was also playing hockey, soccer, and Little League. We had school events and play dates with his friends to work in. Then there were the family holidays like Christmas, Easter, Thanksgiving, and the Fourth of July.

Weekends were packed full to bursting with trips for the racing, sporting events, family camping, and beach trips.

Every minute was booked.

When you are living life at that pace, you don't have a clue what milk costs or what gas costs. You quickly pull in and grab it, thinking, *Whatever. I don't have time to think about the price.* Health? You take it for granted. You are trying to keep so many balls in the air, there's no time to stop and think . . . it was "extreme living." But Aaron and I and everybody in our circles were into extreme. We craved it.

I was barreling down the path of my life paying no attention whatsoever to my soul. If your soul can't get your attention, it uses other means.

First, it tries emotion: stress, anxiety, unhappiness.

Then, it turns to your body.

Into this mix, Aaron and I dropped a huge project. During the spring and summer of 1992, we were working with a contractor to build a custom-designed 4,200-square-foot house with four bathrooms on five wooded acres. The land had a gorgeous view of the river and valley below—and a stream running through it, no less.

As anyone who has built a house will tell you, it takes a lot of work. And a lot of money. We began to wonder if we would be able to afford to live in our house when it was finally finished. The house project felt like a monster baby that couldn't get fed fast enough. We'd throw large amounts of money at it, turn around and it needed to be fed cash again. *Hey! Didn't I just feed you?*

Aaron and I had arranged with the building contractor to do as much of the work as we were able (and skilled enough) to do. That was the only way we could afford it. We came home from our full-time jobs, and worked on the house every night and whenever else we could find a few spare minutes.

I remember Aaron sitting on a makeshift scaffolding in the nearly pitch-black living room and foyer one night at 1:30 a.m. The foyer had a twenty-five-foot ceiling and only a small portion of the wall could be illuminated with our puny amateur lights. We had to get the walls painted before morning. The next round of subcontractors wouldn't be able to do the work they needed to do if we didn't finish. We had headed here right after work, put seven-year-old Colin to bed on a pallet in one of the unfinished bedrooms, and rolled up our sleeves. The paint from the compressor Aaron was using kept getting into his contact lenses even though he was wearing goggles. We pushed and cursed our way through most of the night, then caught a few hours of sleep before we started our day jobs the next morning. This was typical.

We both became accustomed to constant exhaustion.

In the middle of needing money to feed the incessantly hungry house project, I was told that my position at the local county courthouse might be cut due to budget constraints. I was a particular judge's court stenographer and I loved working with him. It was up to the County Council whether my job with him would continue. I anxiously awaited each of their biweekly meetings where the existence of my position was one of the scheduled issues to be addressed. Each session, the future of my job position got pushed to the next meeting's agenda.

The ironic thing was: *I never actually lost my job.* I was just kept on tenterhooks, labeled as a temporary contract employee, waiting for the next session when the County Council might ax my position. It never happened. But the emotional effect penetrated deep.

I couldn't understand why I wasn't happy. I was living the American dream. I had a great son and a devoted husband. My dream house was on the way. I had a career I loved and in which I commanded respect.

I also was regularly working eighty-hour weeks for the courthouse, commuting to work in terrible traffic, running a household, raising a seven-year-old, preserving my marriage, and cleaning the building site for the new house . . . all of this . . . every . . . day.

Still, I didn't get it. I couldn't understand how someone with a life this idyllic could feel so bad.

Why did I need sleeping pills to keep my mind from running over and over my worries all night long? Why was I putting on weight because I couldn't resist the comfort of sugar, salt, and deep-fried foods? Why did each setback on the house send me into an internal maelstrom of irritation and aggravation with no peace in sight?

I had been raised in a very religious household. My parents were both practicing Roman Catholics. I'd gone to Catholic schools, married a Catholic man, and baptized my baby Catholic. But I had always felt like a square peg tapped into a round hole in the church pew. A square peg wearing a plaid skirt, knee socks, and penny loafers complete with a shiny penny. It never occurred to me to turn to God in hard times—God wasn't someone at our beck and call. Who was I to ask the Almighty for help with my problems? (Problems I had no doubt brought on myself, by the way.) You pull yourself up by your own bootstraps—that's what I'd been taught—and don't go bothering God with your puny self-created troubles. Who do you think you are?

So I went on bootstrapping it.

You learn so many fascinating things when you're a court stenographer. I remember the day an oncologist testified that there was one factor that showed up in 95 percent of the cases where people develop cancer: There was always a sustained major stress in their life the year before the cancer grew to be life-threatening.

"Stress creates disease," the oncologist stated. "Physical or emotional—take your pick. If you really want to give cancer a fighting chance, try both for good measure."

With the combination of the physical demands of the house project and the emotional stress of possibly losing my job, I was unconsciously creating the perfect breeding ground for disease. And, unbeknownst to me, I had a disease ready and waiting.

The hepatitis C was replicating exponentially in my emotionally stressed and physically exhausted body. I was too busy to notice how I felt. More and more hep C organisms moved in to hiding places in my body. They hid in cells in my spine, my brain, my kidneys—there are endless places to play hide-n-seek for the hep C virus—but especially in my liver. The hep C loved my liver! The liver is hepatitis C's favorite place to move in, set up housekeeping, put its feet up and say, "This is my territory now. I now declare this 'Camp Hep C.'"

All the while, I had no idea that I was in a fight for survival. I didn't notice the warning signs. Or I was too busy to give them any weight.

So I'm a little run down. Who wouldn't be?

I was typing up court transcripts on my lunch hours, picking up debris and sweeping floors at the construction site every night, shopping for dinner, running a bath for my seven-year-old—I had no boundaries and no limits. I was numb to my body and constantly ignored its needs. For example, I remember feeding myself a nonstop stream of caramels in order to pull an all-nighter and finish a difficult transcription job for the next day.

We put the house we were living in on the market. There was no telling how long it would take to sell, and we would need the money after moving into our new house. Unexpectedly, it sold in a flash. The buyers wanted to move in within a month and our new home wasn't anywhere near ready to be occupied. The walls were hardly up.

A good friend came to the rescue and generously offered his sixteen-foot camper for us to use in the interim. Whew! He did warn us that the old abandoned camper was moldy and not in good shape but it would at least provide a roof over our heads. We gratefully accepted and moved into it with a few boxes of our summer clothing. *It's only for a few weeks, right?*

Fellow home-builders—you know this scenario well. The house project took longer than we expected.

We had moved into the camper in the middle of summer, thinking it would be a four- to six-week stay. But weeks dragged into months. As fall progressed, we good-naturedly dug through the boxes in storage to find long-sleeved shirts, gloves, and jackets to get us through the colder months descending upon us. Still, the 4,200-square-foot home was not anywhere near completion. There was one delay and complication after another.

Living in that camper became more challenging as the weather became cold and wet. One morning, as I was putting on my make-up, I felt something squishier than usual under my feet. Here I am in a sixteen-foot camper trying to make myself presentable for a courtroom environment. I pretzeled into a shape that allowed me to look closely at the bathroom carpet. Mushrooms! Honest to God, there were mushrooms growing in the damp, moldy bathroom carpet.

Just hang in there. It'll only be a little longer. We're creating our dream. We're almost there.

Unbeknownst to me, hepatitis C continued homesteading my body while I was distracted finishing the new house. I had grown accustomed to the now constant fatigue and going to bed exhausted every night. One day I contracted a respiratory cold that wouldn't go away. I figured I was having a hard time kicking it because I was living in such damp quarters in the camper, sleeping a few feet from fungi-growing carpet.

But it got real serious, real fast.

3

AN ARM FULL OF SCARS

Late one night I collapsed and Aaron rushed me to the hospital. From my perspective, one week I had been an active, competent, thirty-eight-year-old working mother and the next week I was in a hospital bed fighting for my life.

That's what it seemed like.

That was my perception. But of course that wasn't what had happened at all.

Remember the oncologist's testimony: Physical exhaustion plus emotional stress equals disease. I had done everything I could to invite disaster. I had ignored my every need. I was last on the list. I didn't count. And now I had reached the end of the path that I had been walking for so long. It was inevitable.

At that time medical science had not identified the existence of hepatitis C. They had no idea what was destroying my internal organs. All they knew was that my liver and kidneys were shutting down and that my head cold had turned to bronchitis headed for pneumonia.

As sick as I was, I had enough awareness of my surroundings to see the fear on my doctors' faces as they watched a healthy young mother slipping away from their healing grasp.

My husband visited me each night. One evening he came in with a big smile all ready for me, and as soon as he saw me, his face trembled uncontrollably and the tears started pouring down his cheeks. I must have looked pretty bad.

He quickly explained the tears away, saying it was because he missed me so much. I played along and pretended that he wasn't afraid I was dying. But I knew he was scared . . . and so was I. Actually, I'm not sure which was harder, the tears or the nights he feigned cheery optimism as he gave my pale, weak body a hug and tried not to break down again.

Now I prayed.

There are no atheists in foxholes, after all. But I still didn't feel God's presence. Maybe, deep down, I didn't think I deserved it.

Aaron's mom, my sweet mother-in-law, Tillie McConnell, was a very devoted Catholic. She went to church every day of her life as far as I know. One evening while I was in the hospital, she was praying on her patio looking out over the ocean in California and crying because she was so worried. "Mother Mary, Mother of Mercy. Our life, our sweetness, and our hope . . ."

Then she heard a voice in her head. Such a thing had never happened to her before.

The voice said, *She'll be all right.*

Tillie called Aaron and me the next day to tell us about it. We knew how devoted and spiritual Tillie was, so we took the message to heart. It gave us some comfort. *She'll be all right.* We reminded each other of that message whenever it didn't look as if I would live.

My circle of doctors widened as the doctors who were currently working on me brought in more and more colleagues and specialists. Still, they were perplexed. No one seemed to know why I was slipping away so fast. None of the treatments were working.

Unsure what was wrong with me, they had placed me in the hospital where they originally thought I might need to be—the cancer ward. I could see the lights across the hall late into the night as radiation therapy was administered around the clock to cancer patients. *Was that where I was headed?*

One of the experts called in was a kidney specialist named Dr. Schultz. He had a thick German accent that distinguished him for me from the many doctors who shuffled in and out of my room. I wasn't always lucid during doctor visits, but I do remember the day that Dr. Schultz came in very excited.

"I believe I know what is wrong with you," he exclaimed in his heavy accent.

He was smiling broadly. *Finally, some good news.*

"Last week I attended a symposium on Non-A/Non-B hepatitis," he told me. "We have discovered a strain of hepatitis that is not hepatitis A or hepatitis B. It is a new strain, so new that it has not even been named yet. But your symptoms match the description for this new hepatitis perfectly." (Of course, it was this new strain that would later be called hepatitis C.)

You have probably guessed that, since they didn't have a name for it, they didn't have a cure. They didn't even have a standard treatment. Hepatitis C was often fatal at that time, usually due to severe liver damage. But it also attacked the other organs—hep C is open-minded that way. It'll eat anything.

Dr. Schultz was convinced I had this new strain of hepatitis. He knew that I had sustained quite a bit of damage and that among other problems I had severely damaged kidneys.

"Not to worry," said Dr. Schultz. He enthusiastically pulled up the sleeve of his long-sleeved white shirt and displayed an arm pocked with scars from hundreds of needles inserted into his veins. "I have been on kidney dialysis for years."

I know he was trying to encourage me, but honestly—that horribly scarred arm shocked the hell out of me.

Dr. Schultz remained ebullient, however. They finally knew what was wrong with me, and they could try to treat it. Instead of slipping quietly away in this hospital bed, I now stood a chance of survival.

Eventually I was sent to the liver research clinic at a large hospital in Seattle. It had some of the leading researchers for liver disease in the country. I saw a top-notch doctor named Dr. David Dahl. He was also extraordinarily personable. I learned all about his kids and his hobbies during our weekly visits.

One day I was talking with him and, suddenly, I needed to vomit (one of the side effects of hepatitis C). He casually reached over, grabbed the metal wastebasket from beside his desk and handed it to me. I vomited inside the metal container and handed it back to him apologetically. He never skipped a beat. He kept talking with straight eye contact, unflinching. I got the impression that many of his patients vomited in his wastebasket during consultations. I have to admit, he made what would have been an embarrassing situation seem totally natural.

Dr. Dahl explained that the only thing they could offer me, at this early stage in their research, was the use of a cancer-fighting drug, which they would be using on me in an experimental way. The drug was Interferon, a drug aimed at boosting the immune system. I would be taking very high doses mixed with other drugs they were testing—a cocktail that would hopefully keep the hep C at bay. The hep C monster had come out of the basement and we had to coax it back in and shut the door. Interferon had been used successfully to fight leukemia. They were going to see how it did with hepatitis C.

He told me that from what they knew at that time, there was no cure. Once hepatitis C set up house inside you, it never left. The best we could hope for was that we could get it to become a better-mannered roommate, meaning that we could convince the hep C not to kill me.

Unfortunately (there seemed to be so many of those "unfortunatelys"), there were a lot of bad side effects to this experimental drug mixture. Very few patients could endure the side effects of this particular Interferon cocktail for a single six-month course. Even fewer could take more than one course.

I would take whatever slim chance I could get.

4

ONE CRASH
IS NOT ENOUGH

I was sitting on the closed toilet seat in the bathroom of our dream home staring at my scarred thigh, trying to get up the courage to jab myself one more time. After the injection, I would feel severe flu-like symptoms throughout the night and well into the next day. Fever, headache, muscle pain, nausea, and diarrhea. The worst was the fatigue, the constant debilitating fatigue. By the time I started to feel a little better, it would be time to give myself another shot.

Some days I could sit there for almost an hour, before working up enough nerve to jab myself.

The trick was not to pause like this and think about it.

Too late.

My vitality, how good or bad I felt, had become defined by what day of the week it was. I dreaded Mondays, Wednesdays, and Fridays. Those were the days I had to give myself the shots that were keeping me alive while at the same time costing me my well-being.

Sundays offered a bit of relief. On Sundays the side effects of my life-saving drug had worn off enough to give me a few hours of feeling half-human. It was that one day a week of almost-feeling-good that gave me something to look forward to.

I was told this would go on for the rest of my life. There was no cure. My greatest hope was that the medicine would continue to work for me and that, maybe, someday they would find a cure for hepatitis C.

As bad as the side effects of the Interferon were, it worked. It kept the hepatitis C at bay. I was able to function again. I was able to go back to work. I was able to return to my family life. I just felt perpetually terrible.

One night after I began the Interferon, I couldn't sleep for the muscle pain, and I was standing at our fireplace looking at a picture of our sweet, precocious son taken not long before. It was January of 1993 and I had just taken down the Christmas decorations. I had managed to keep the family going on an almost normal keel through Christmas, and Colin was doing well. He was a happy, buoyant, just generally great kid.

Aaron and I had built a gorgeous home. Yes, it had been finished in the fall of 1992 and we had moved in. I loved it. Built like a zigzag, it had interesting angles and floor-to-ceiling windows looking out over the valley and the river below. I had decorated it as I had originally planned, sewing curtains and painting decorative trim and putting up wallpaper. How I did all that while injecting my experimental Interferon blend and working full time, I don't know.

Now in the middle of the night, with the rest of the house sleeping, I stood at the mantel, looking at my seven-year-old son's picture. There he was in his uniform, hands deliberately posed on top of a soccer ball, sporting a sweet innocent grin missing a tooth front and center. I thought about my life at that age. How much did I remember of my mother at age seven?

The only strong memory I had of age seven was that I had been sick on Valentine's Day and hadn't been able to go to the class party and receive my valentines. I didn't remember my teacher.

I didn't remember what my mother looked like.

I knew in my heart that Colin would be too young to remember me if I died right now. He wouldn't know so many things about me: that I loved frosting, that I was passionate about animals, that I was lousy at math, was always upbeat, hated to cook, and loved to be outside. He wouldn't remember that, although I was fearless in many ways, I was scared to death of sledding. He was too young to remember all the things I wanted to teach him about life: how to extend forgiveness to those who have hurt you, how to carefully place a bug outside without harming it, how to find humor in the face of adversity, how to be polite and respectful to the elderly . . . so many things I wanted to teach him. He wouldn't have enough memories to sustain him for life.

I could hear him saying, "My mom? I didn't really know my mom. She died when I was young."

My chances were not good. I knew that. I probably wouldn't live to see him get married, let alone hold his children in my arms. But I wanted to at least survive long enough to ensure that Colin would remember me. I wanted him to know who I was. I wanted to give him the gifts that a mother passes on to her child, the important ones, the lasting ones. It was this that kept me going, that made me tenacious in finding answers and staying alive.

When I arrived for the meeting of my Hepatitis Support Group three years later, Colin was ten. It was 1995. I had made it through three more years.

I leaned over to the woman next to me and asked, "Where's Judy tonight?"

"She didn't make it," she whispered back. The meeting was starting. "Oh."

Something in the tone communicated clearly that the woman didn't just mean Judy couldn't come to the Hepatitis Support Group meeting that night. She meant Judy didn't make it period. She had died.

I looked around the circle of fellow survivors on folding chairs with a pleasant, interested mask plastered to my face. An enthusiastic woman was saying she had been trying milk thistle and kombucha mushroom tea. At that time I gave no weight to herbs and potions. Alternative medicine meant nothing to me. And anyway, I didn't really hear her. Even though I had an encouraging smile on my face, I had a hollow void behind my breastbone: *Another member of my monthly support group had died.*

The only thing I could think was, *I'm still alive. I'm beating the odds. Why?*

The support group was a band of highly intelligent survivors determined to fight hep C with everything available to them. I was impressed with the depth of their knowledge, not only about the disease itself, but about future treatments and who was doing what research in which countries. Yet every few months there was one less person who showed up because they had died. Despite their valiant and courageous efforts to survive, some of them died anyway. These people weren't just hepatitis C *statistics* to me. (Cue announcer: "Yesterday in its annual report, the CDC reported 3,000 deaths associated with the hepatitis C virus last year.") These were real people that I could put a face to—*friends.* I had shared information and laughs and experiences with them. And one by one, we kept losing them.

Yet, I still survived.

Why?

It started raising questions in my mind.

Was it just luck? I had never been one to win a raffle. Even if I held 98 of the 100 tickets for the cake raffle in my sweaty hand, I could pretty much guarantee I was not going to be eating any carrot cake that night. I didn't buy lottery tickets for that reason. And yet, I had survived for three years. I had been unbelievably lucky. Or had I?

As I sat in this meeting, I started to realize that it was one unlikely coincidence after another that had kept me alive: Dr. Schultz happened to have been called in to treat me, and he happened to attend a symposium on hepatitis C the next week. I happened to have a disease for which the most advanced research in the country was being done right here in Seattle. They happened to be researching an experimental treatment that would work for me. I happened to qualify to be a candidate for the experimental group. I happened to be one of the 25 percent of patients for whom the Interferon treatment had been effective. I succeeded again with the second round of Interferon treatment—even though it was only effective for 25 percent of the remaining 25 percent of patients. And the next round . . . and the next. For three years.

Maybe I *should* start buying lottery tickets.

Or maybe something besides luck was at work here.

I began to ask myself: *Is there a spiritual side of life? Is there a spiritual purpose to it?* Everyone alive at this moment was going to die sometime. We all die. Was there any kind of sense as to when? Maybe everyone alive has something they need to accomplish and they are not going to be leaving one minute before they do what they came here to do. Was the reason I survived because my life's mission had not been completed?

So many synchronicities. How could it be just random?

If life and death were not random, if there was any kind of order or plan to the universe, then did that mean there was a divine intelligence arranging things? Not a distant, judgmental, condemning God, but a Creator who was present to us and cared about our life's purpose. A higher consciousness who knew us and kept track of the events in all our lives.

If that was true, what should I do about it?

This is when the questions first started prodding me. Did I do anything about it? Did I start looking for spiritual answers in new places? Start praying, start meditating, start talking to people, start opening to messages from my soul—even just a little?

Well . . . life settled into its old whirlwind of responsibilities. I was working full time again. I had to keep my job at the courthouse, in spite of the side effects of the Interferon mixture, because my medications were costing more than $1,000 a month—I had to have medical insurance. I needed to get up at 4:30 a.m. to get Colin to hockey practice on time. Christmas cookies needed to be baked for the radio-controlled car racing club bake sale. I think the dog needed a flea bath and—need I say more?

A life-threatening illness had crashed into my life to direct me onto a different spiritual path.

Evidently, one crash was not enough.

5

GOOD-BYE MEMORY

The average hepatitis C patient at my clinic took the Interferon compound in the dosages I was taking it for six months max. I took it for five *years*. From the summer of 1993 to the spring of 1998. Colin was thirteen. I'd given him the presence of his mother for five more years.

On top of the flu-like symptoms, like aches, chills, and shaking, my body started exhibiting other symptoms toward the end of 1997.

My heart labored; my blood pounded in my ears. *Ignore it.*

My lungs felt constricted; I couldn't get my breath. *Move slower.*

My kidneys hurt; I had to urinate every half hour. *Where's the nearest ladies' room?*

My head ached, sometimes for days at a time. *Work through the pain, girl. It's not that bad.*

Finally, I was having trouble seeing. When I pulled my eyelids to the side, I could clearly see pockets of swelling. *Well . . . eat less salt. Try to get more rest. Exercise, no matter how exhausted you feel. Stay positive. Don't dwell on the medical situation. Just keep going.*

I kept on working, taking care of the family, holding down my job, managing special events . . . until I couldn't.

One Friday morning in May of 1998, I couldn't get up from my bed. I couldn't think. I couldn't finish a sentence. I couldn't see. And I couldn't get in to see my specialists at the hepatitis clinic until Monday.

The following Monday in the examination room, I turned the lights off because they hurt my head and eyes so badly. I lay down on the table, waiting for the doctor. I couldn't get in to see my regular doctor at the clinic, so another doctor was going to evaluate my trouble. I knew all the doctors at the clinic were experts, some of the foremost experts in the country. I was in good hands.

When he arrived and turned the lights on, he looked at my chart, then at me with wonder, then back at my chart. "Well, you hold the record," he said.

I struggled to a sitting position. "Excuse me?"

"I've never seen a patient take this Interferon mix at these dosages as long as you have. Normally, our test subjects can take this particular prescription for three to six months. Five years? It's a new planetary record. With these symptoms, we have to discontinue. I can't believe you've held out this long."

"But what about my hep C? The Interferon is the only thing keeping me alive."

"You have basically had a severe reaction to the drug. With these symptoms . . . involvement of the heart, the lungs, the kidneys . . . and I think you may also be experiencing intracranial pressure, inflammation that is affecting your brain . . ." He paused looking at the chart. "You have to stop taking the Interferon."

"What else can I take?"

"For the hepatitis C?"

"Yes."

"There is no medication for it that doesn't involve Interferon in some form. Now that you have had a reaction to the drug, reducing the dosage isn't even an option. You must stop taking it in any quantity."

"Then . . ." Before I could think of what to say, he went on.

"Have you seen a neurologist?"

I shook my head.

"I want you to make an appointment right away. I can give you the name of someone if you don't already have a neurologist. And I want you to call them immediately and get an appointment. I'm very concerned about your confusion and memory loss."

"Memory loss?"

"According to the nurse, you were having trouble speaking and remembering words."

"Yes."

"Well, we're concerned about that."

"What about my breathing and my heartbeat . . ."

"Without the Interferon, those symptoms should subside. They should return to normal fairly quickly. You're having an allergic reaction. Your body is rejecting the drug. Once you stop the medicine, the inflammation will decrease and your breathing and heartbeat should go back to normal within a few days. Contact us right away if they don't. You'll need to rest of course. I suggest you rest for at least three months."

He didn't pause at my half-laugh.

"I am more concerned about your memory," he continued. "I want you to make an appointment with the neurologist right away."

What I didn't know was that my brain had been deeply affected by the inflammation. They knew that given time my organs could recover from their allergic reaction to the drugs. But my cognitive function and memory were different. The concern was that the brain damage was permanent.

"But what about the hepatitis?"

"Rest. Eat well. Stay away from heavy fats. Come back in three months and we'll run the blood tests again. Check the liver function."

I nodded dumbly. What else could I say?

And so I was sent home from the clinic—wearing the slippers and pajamas I'd arrived in—to do the best I could.

Without any treatment for the hepatitis C and with the damage from the Interferon, I became virtually bedridden. I fitfully slept twenty or more hours a day. I had pain in strange places, mostly in my joints and muscles. Massive migraine-like headaches came and went. I had to get up and go to the bathroom every half hour.

Aaron and I tried to continue sleeping together, but now, if he touched a painful place on my body in the night, I woke up. He wanted me to be able to rest the many hours I needed to in order to recover. With my frequent bathroom trips, I was waking him up all night long too. I felt terrible about that because Aaron had to get up at 5:00 a.m. to make the long commute to the marina that he managed in Seattle.

So I moved to a bed in our guest room. *It'll only be until I get better.*

Over the next two years, that bed in the guest room became the center for family gatherings. Since I couldn't leave it, the family came to me as they arrived home. We would chat about their day, eat, laugh, and plan our lives on that bed. Even the dog and the cat joined the pile.

I did see the recommended neurologist and dozens of other doctors. I was incredibly tenacious about finding a way to recover, but I was in bad shape. I had, in fact, sustained considerable brain damage. My short-term memory was horribly impaired. And there was no guarantee of recovery. I finally found a neurologist that became my primary doctor. He was a wonderful, patient, and compassionate man. He was able to identify the parts of my cognitive functioning that had been damaged and help me track the slow, slow, slow improvement.

For example, one day I remembered that the little white thing on the bathroom counter (the cap I had removed moments before) could be used to close up the toothpaste tube. "So that's how the toothpaste stays in the tube!" I said.

Yes, it was bad.

I had lost a lot of my long-term memories. Particularly, the years preceding the allergic reaction. Colin became used to me saying, "I'm sorry, I don't remember that," about things we had done together as a family.

But it was the loss of my short-term memory function that was the most distressing. I couldn't finish a sentence because I forgot what I was talking about. I would return a phone call twice because I couldn't remember that I had just called them. When I was putting on my clothes, I couldn't remember if the tag went in the front or the back. When I tried to read, I had to read the same words over and over and over. I couldn't remember what I wanted to jot down (in order to remember it) long enough to jot it down.

As a court stenographer, I had prided myself on the perfection of my grammar and spelling. Now I couldn't for the life of me figure out how to spell "went" and "how."

Good-bye job at the courthouse. Good-bye career as a court stenographer. Yes, you have to have a functioning memory to report court proceedings verbatim.

Meanwhile, I tenaciously sought answers for both the hepatitis C and the mental and physical damage from my reaction to the Interferon. As I went from one specialist to another, it became increasingly clear that I had been shuffled out the back door by Western medicine. Despite their desire to help, there seemed to be nothing they could offer me. I had plumbed the depths of their little black bag.

Divine Spirit was pushing me into the unknown and unknowable, into the mysteries of the universe, in a big way.

6

A VISIT WITH
GRANDPA HOMER

When you are desperate for answers, you can find yourself pursuing them in the most unlikely places. That's what I was thinking as I mounted the porch of a consultant named Deirdre. I was there on the advice of a friend who told me Deirdre had been able to help her improve her health. My friend had said, "She just knows things."

The house was in an upscale neighborhood, and her yard was well landscaped with a lush lawn and a large front porch. *Wow,* I thought. *This is a really nice place. Whatever she does, she must be well respect—.*

Then I saw the gargoyles guarding the front door.

It was late in 1999, about a year after I was no longer able to take Interferon. My health wasn't good, but my mind had recovered enough to be able to drive myself to this appointment, at least. I was still alive. I was surviving the hepatitis for the time being. But I hadn't been able to return to work or to taking care of my family. Every minute I felt tired to my marrow, and I was in bed twenty hours a day. During every hour I could be awake and active, I was relentlessly searching for a path back to health. Evidently, the search was taking me to some weird places.

The gargoyles I was contemplating were two-foot-tall cement statues of demons with hollowed out eyes and gaping mouths. Coming from my Midwest conservative Roman Catholic background, I wondered what I had gotten myself into. There are certain images that were downright scary for me, and howling fanged monsters was one of them. But I had gone down every alley to try to recover my health. I was up for anything that might actually work. So I brushed aside my fears and rang the doorbell.

The woman who had recommended Deirdre was the mother of one of my son's friends. Her name was Jen, and she and I had something more in common than hockey-playing teenage boys. We both shared another newly discovered illness: fibromyalgia.

My poor body had been so whacked out of balance, it developed yet another set of symptoms.

After my primary doctor had established I was no longer suffering an immune reaction to the Interferon, I was left with some symptoms that weren't necessarily typical of hepatitis alone. I had muscle pain all over, severe fatigue, sleeplessness, and sensitivity to light, noise, and cold. Those were a few of the baffling symptoms. Searching in the library, I found an illness that exhibited most of the symptoms I had. It had been named fibromyalgia. I took the question to my doctor and he confirmed the diagnosis. He told me he used two criteria in addition to my bucketful of symptoms: "1) widespread pain for at least three months in three quadrants of the body, and 2) abnormal sensitivity to palpation in at least 11 of 18 specific tender points."

As I said, Jen was also struggling with fibromyalgia. She told me about seeing a consultant who had been very helpful. She said Deirdre was intuitive, that she had told Jen things about her health, what was affecting it, and what could improve it. Following Deirdre's advice, Jen had gotten a lot better. *A consultant who was intuitive? What was that?*

Jen said Deirdre was well respected and that she had many well-off clients, including some in Hollywood. I knew Jen was well educated and careful about her medical care. I also knew she was married to a successful lawyer. Surely, if there was anything questionable about

Deirdre, Jen would never have recommended her. And Jen was so positive Deirdre had helped her with her fibromyalgia. A little flame of hope sprang up in me.

So I made an appointment and went.

I walked up onto Deirdre's porch committed to keeping an open mind.

When Deirdre answered the door, her appearance reassured me. She was an elegantly dressed brunette with a wide smile and a voice like melted chocolate. Her rich, deep laugh put me instantly at ease. She ushered me into a living room decorated with the most unusual furnishings and lovely art. I found it all very stylish and incredibly creative. Even though everything was oversized, exaggerated, richly colored and textured, the effect was still elegant and comfortable.

When I asked to use the rest room, I was blown away by the bathroom walls. They were textured with what looked like crinkled tissue paper, lacquered and painted in teal and gold and green. Like the rest of the house, the effect was very luxurious and soothing at the same time. I found out later some of her clients were movie set designers and they gave her decorating tips.

I was very intrigued by this woman as she sat down cross-legged in a gigantic purple chair across from me. She didn't start off by asking me any questions. She simply said, "So . . . I'm an intuitive."

I nodded, even though I really had no idea what that meant.

"People call me when they're stuck and need a little help understanding what's going on. I'll need to hold something from you like a piece of jewelry. Something that carries your energy. That'll help tell me your story."

How bizarre, I thought. *Oh well, I'm here now.*

I'm not normally much for jewelry but I was wearing a watch. (I'm not big on jewelry, but I'm big on time.)

She took my watch, held it in both hands, and raised her eyes above my head. She was focusing as if she were watching a movie playing out over my head. She began talking very fast.

She started by telling me about the house in which I was living and my husband and son. She went into the minutest detail. I had told this woman nothing about my life. Could Jen have told her these things? It didn't seem likely Jen had wasted her consultation time describing the octagonal-shaped bathroom sink in my house and my husband's love of mango-topped halibut. So how could Deirdre know these things about me?

Then, Deirdre began to describe in eerie detail the prescription drugs I was taking. There were fourteen at the time. She discussed the purpose each was intended to have and the side effects they were having on my body. She went on to tell me the number of doctors helping me (there were four I was seeing) and what they looked like and what their personalities were like.

One of the doctors treating me at the time was a bit egotistical. "The primary doctor treating you is tall with dark hair and dark eyes," she said. "He's very handsome and he knows it." She went on to describe him and his mannerisms perfectly. Chuckling to myself, I thought, *Boy, you just nailed him.*

When I realized she knew as much about my health care as I did, I sat up and started paying attention.

"How are you able to know these things?" I asked. Just friendly.

"What I see in my mind's eye is like a wall of nine television screens with different scenes playing in each one. Each screen holds a different story of your life. I choose whichever channel I want to look at and follow the story out."

We were interrupted by the doorbell—a very unusual-sounding doorbell. Nothing in this place was ordinary; it was all fascinating. A delivery man was at the door with a huge bouquet of yellow roses. Deirdre glowed with pleasure as she placed them in the center of her dining room table.

"Those are gorgeous," I said. "Who are they from?" I've always been unabashed about my nosiness.

"Oh." She hesitated briefly, while humility battled girlish

enjoyment. "They're from a director in Hollywood who I helped last week." Apparently, she really did have Hollywood clients.

She sat back down in the chair across from me and resumed focusing again on my "screens." Her accuracy and the amount of detail astounded me. She knew things about me there was no imaginable way she could possibly know. She told me about my five siblings and that I was raised in the Midwest among rows of cornfields.

Up to now Deirdre had been talking very fast. It was like she could hardly keep up with the reel being played on the screen in front of her. But suddenly, she became quiet, almost as if she were listening to someone. What she said next rocked my world.

"Your grandfather is here with us," she said.

"My grandfather?" I asked, looking around as if I might see him. The hair on my arms was standing on end. This was very weird.

"Yes, Homer. He loves you very much."

I was shocked and immediately skeptical. What was going on here? How could she know about my father's father, Homer? How could she even know his name? He had died twenty years ago from cancer. Although I had loved him dearly, I hadn't thought about him in years.

Deirdre was unfazed by my dead grandfather appearing to her. I couldn't see or hear him but apparently he was carrying on quite a conversation with her. She paused, as if listening. Then she turned to me, leaned forward, and said, "Homer says you were his favorite grandchild."

I had loved my grandfather and knew we had a special bond, but he had seemed to love all his grandchildren equally. I had never felt like he singled me out. Although, now that I thought about it, of all ten grandchildren, I was the only one to whom he had ever loaned money, so far as I knew. The loan had enabled me to finish college.

Still, I was skeptical about this Homer thing. "Are you sure it's Grandpa Homer?"

"Yeah," Deirdre replied. "He says he used to farm years ago."

"I don't think so," I said. I didn't remember ever hearing that he farmed. As far as I knew, he'd been a factory worker all his life. "Are you sure you've got the right grandfather?"

"That's what he's telling me." Deirdre was unflappable. "He wants you to know: You're on the right track. Keep going."

The hour flew by as Deirdre gave me more messages from Homer and information about how I could get better. For example, she told me about some foods she thought would help me. Then she gave me a business card with the phone number of a friend of hers who was a naturopathic doctor. Deirdre felt confident this naturopath would be able to get me back on my feet again. When it was time to leave, I thanked her for this fascinating hour, shook her hand, and walked outside.

There were two women with excitement etched on their faces sitting on the top step of the porch—gargoyles on either side of them. Deirdre boomed a welcoming hello as she embraced them one at a time and ushered them inside.

Later that evening, I called my dad back in Illinois. We had a nice conversation, catching up on the latest news with each other. As we were ready to hang up, I said, "Dad, did Grandpa Homer ever farm?"

He paused, searching his memory, and then said, "Yeah, when he was really young. I'd forgotten all about it. I don't think your mother even knows that. Why on Earth would you ask?"

Without disclosing that I was checking the validity of an etheric visitation, I asked him other questions. Dad confirmed everything Deirdre had said to me about my grandfather.

But he had died more than twenty years ago! How could this woman have known things I didn't even know myself—unless she were talking directly to Homer? I was determined to find the answer to that question.

7
HERBS AND POTIONS AFTER ALL

Before a week had gone by, I went to see the naturopath Deirdre had recommended: Dr. Emily Giles. The term *naturopath* was new to me. I wasn't sure what that meant or what a naturopathic doctor did. All I knew was Deirdre seemed to have uncanny abilities, and she had been sure Dr. Giles could help me.

Dr. Giles shared an office with other health practitioners in a nearby town. After Deirdre's unusual workplace, I wasn't sure what to expect. When I arrived I saw this was a normal medical environment. Dr. Giles' office looked pretty much like any other doctor's office, with a waiting room and a receptionist.

Dr. Giles came out to greet me—a willowy green-eyed woman with a cap of tousled dark curls and a friendly, confident handshake.

She took me to her sunny corner office. Again, nothing all that strange: a small desk, an examination table, and an overstuffed book-shelf. Well, maybe the vining plant hanging in the corner was a little more lush than you would see in most examination rooms. And there were considerably more glass-fronted shelves lining the walls than in other doctors' offices. Still, the questions she asked me as I sat across from her at the wooden desk were familiar. I settled into my usual spiel—after an entire year of seeing one specialist after another, I had the recitation of my symptoms down pat.

The standard medical methods and approaches stopped there.

She had me get on the examination table and lie down fully clothed on my back. I stared at the flower designs she had painted on the ceiling above the table. Then, she held her hands about eight inches above me, palms down. Without touching me, she moved her hands over the entire length of my body, as if she were feeling something in the air. This took about five minutes, maybe a little longer. Then silence.

She was concentrating hard, and I didn't want to interrupt her thoughts with any questions. She picked up a flat white plastic tray and moved over to the shelves. I continued to lie there. I noticed for the first time the vast array of bottles behind those glass doors. They seemed to contain . . . what? Herbs, capsules, potions? It looked like she kept her pharmacy right here in the office.

She had been silent during the exam, but now I could hear her muttering under her breath, "Ah yes, a little bit of this. Does your body want that? No. This? No. This? Ah, yes! This is the one. But I'm missing . . . what, what, what . . . here it is!"

I tilted my head so I could watch her. This curious woman was holding her hand out to the shelves. She was feeling in the air in front of the shelves just as she had felt in the air over my body. As she talked she would occasionally grab a bottle and put it in the tray.

She continued to put different medicines into the tray. Finally, she brought the tray filled with bottles over to me. As I continued to lie there, she held the small white plastic bin suspended about eight inches above my heart and considered. Not as if she was considering what was in the tray, but as if she was *having a silent conversation* with what was in the tray.

"This is it," she finally said.

Dr. Giles then explained which herbs and supplements I was to take, how often, and when. I was going home with about six bottles of strange-sounding herbs—all unfamiliar to me but not entirely odd in their appearance.

"Come back next week and we'll see how you're doing."

I scheduled my next appointment with my arms stocked with bottles and went home mystified as to what had just happened. The process was unconventional—not sinister, but different.

Dr. Giles had never once touched my body during the examination and yet she seemed to have a clear and confident idea of what was wrong with me and what I needed to take to help heal it. She seemed able to internally scan my body without the aid of instruments.

She used her hands to sense—what?—from my body and from her medicines. It was as if the hundred different bottles on the shelves were speaking to her, telling her which ones to use and how much. It was like she was listening to a radio channel that I couldn't tune in. Well, we would see how "tuned-in" she was.

I went home. I did as she asked. I got better.

I was able to get up for five hours during a day, then six hours, then seven. I was able to do some housework without feeling exhausted. The headaches became less severe and less frequent. I went ten minutes without any body pain at all, then twenty minutes, then a whole afternoon.

I truly didn't understand what she was doing but I wasn't about to stop seeing her. I was getting well. What else mattered? Deirdre had said, "I think this doctor will help you," and I went because it was the only card I had at that time. Fortunately, it turned out it was the only card I needed.

Western medicine had saved me the first time I nearly died. It was Dr. Giles who saved me now. Slowly, without the use of any medical instruments, drugs, or medical tests, using what appeared to be only her instincts and natural homeopathic herbs, Dr. Giles brought me back to life again.

Dr. Giles, it turned out, is a naturopathic doctor with unusual gifts and abilities. I didn't know it at the time, but not all naturopaths operate like this. I didn't realize until much, much later that Dr. Giles knew how to *read* my energy field and *see* internally into my body. She saw the energetic pattern of my body. And she saw the energetic gateways that allowed life force to flow into and out of my body.

The life force of our bodies is called by many different names in other cultures: *prana* in Ayurvedic medicine and *chi* or *qi* or *ki* in various Asian medicine traditions. The energetic gateways for this life force are often called *chakras* (after their Hindu name). The chakras are supposed to open and spin to draw in this life force, to keep it flowing through the energetic pathways of the body and mind, and to keep the spiritual, mental, emotional, and physical health of the body in balance. Dr. Giles could sense these chakras and determine if they were open and spinning or if they were blocked or closed.

All through the winter and spring of 2000, I saw Dr. Giles. We would sit and discuss the emotional components of my illnesses and my need to slow down emotionally and physically. She emphasized my need to take care of myself, eat well, exercise a little but not too strenuously. "Perhaps you might try gentle walking," she said. Then she would repeat the process of scanning my body's energy field with her hands and instinctively knowing which herbs would help unblock the energy and heal me.

At first I was too sick to care what she was doing. But as I got better and started miraculously regaining my health and energy, I was curious about her methods. It seemed so un-intrusive, so easy, so natural. What was she *doing*?

And Deirdre? How could she have known Dr. Giles would help me? How was Deirdre able to describe my four doctors, my fourteen medications, my childhood? And how could she know about Grandpa Homer?

It was pretty hard to deny that Dr. Giles and Deirdre were accessing a reality I had never known existed. What were they seeing that I wasn't? How were they able to communicate with these unseen worlds?

Whatever they were doing, it was working.

They were very quiet about the world they operated in. They never lectured or talked about the "other dimension" of reality. I wanted to know more. It was the first time I looked at the spiritual side of life and asked, *What do they know that I don't?*

I was ready to learn.

When I set out to satisfy my curiosity, I had no idea I was starting out on a path into limitless dimensions that would disassemble my world and remake my life completely.

8

FLYING DOWN
THE PATH

After Dr. Giles started working on me in 1999, all my symptoms started slowly, slowly, slowly to recede. I definitely felt better physically and my memory improved. I was able to read, to drive myself around with more confidence. I still had Post-It Notes up all over the house reminding me of things I mustn't forget (where I hid the birthday presents, for example), but at least I could remember something long enough to put it on a Post-It Note.

It was two steps forward and one step back. I would push my limits and end up in bed for a few days, helpless with fatigue and pain. Then I'd get up and try again and I would be stronger. It was slow progress, but progress it was.

I was getting better and I had no idea why. Deirdre's and Dr. Giles' techniques were a complete mystery. So I set out to solve that mystery. Hah! If I'd only known. I was stepping through a door into another universe with a million paths to explore.

I started by perusing Dr. Giles' bookshelves, and asking her questions about what I saw there. Then, I would find the books at the library, or I would order them, and study them. I read about energy fields and chakras and about other cultures' medical systems. Some of these medical systems had been practiced for thousands of years. I learned there are emotional components to our physical illnesses, that our very thoughts contribute to our healing.

I started reading everything I could get my hands on and listening to books on tape as I drove. I explored writings about the soul and dove with fascination into books like *Echoes of the Soul* by Echo Bodine and *Journey of Souls* by Michael Newton, Ph.D. They talked about how we are souls having a physical experience, not primarily bodies with a soul. I discovered I was an eternal soul! I had never thought about existing before I was born, about making agreements with my parents, my friends, and those I loved to meet in this life. I had never thought about possibly having multiple lives.

As I broadened my reach, I devoured books on the path to enlightenment by the Dalai Lama and others. I studied mindfulness through Eckhart Tolle's *The Power of Now*. I started practicing exercises that were in their books, trying to achieve inner stillness and staying focused in the present moment. Then I discovered books about working with angels and our spirit guides by authors like Dr. Doreen Virtue. It was fascinating.

There was a bookstore in our town that specialized in spiritual, philosophical, and self-healing topics: mind/body/spirit connection, alternative healing modalities, the energetic patterning of our bodies, the extrasensory powers of the mind, and philosophies about time and space. It had a large room for book signings, author talks, meetings, and fairs.

I started attending classes there on developing intuition, how to use telepathy for animal communication, anything they offered.

The more I learned, the more it felt like truth to me.

There were group meditations held in the evenings in the back room. The group leader, Angela, was a beautiful woman with long blond hair and enormous dark-blue eyes. She led a guided meditation, sometimes singing in a clear haunting voice. We would all lie on the floor. I hadn't been so relaxed in years. As instructed, I would try to "see the white light." Everyone else seemed able to see it. Every once in a while, I could barely make out a light in my mind's eye. I noticed when I lay next to a certain man, I felt and saw the light much more, so I would surreptitiously arrange to lie next to him. If he ever clued in I was sponging off his spiritual ability, he never complained. After each of these sessions I would feel much more peaceful and enlivened. So I kept going back.

So much of what I investigated resonated with me. If an idea didn't seem to be something I could accept, I set that investigation aside, no harm done. Meanwhile, I felt like the information I was learning was opening my eyes, my heart, my spirit like the petals of a bud opening to full flower.

One Saturday morning about six months after I had started exploring this new world, Aaron, who had been deep in an aviation magazine all through breakfast, called out to me as I was leaving the house. "Hey Rob, want to go to Chico's for dinner after we watch the boat race today?"

I swiveled. "I won't be at the race today. Remember? I've got that Reiki healing author I'm going to go see speak."

"Huh???" It was that drawn out, rising inflection I hated—like the sound of an ambulance siren starting up. It was an inflection that was unequivocally belittling. An inflection that clearly said, *That nonsense? You're kiddin' me.*

I took a deep breath and sat down facing him on the couch. "Honey? This lecture is important to me. The author doesn't come to our area very often and a lot of people from my meditation group say she's awesome. I want to hear what she has to say."

He raised his eyebrows, sighed, and resumed reading his magazine. "Okay," he huffed. *Conversation ended.*

"Why don't you come with me?"

"Rob, it's not my thing."

"You act like my interest in . . ." What? How would I describe what I was interested in here? "In something that can't be seen . . . something that's behind it all . . . is silly. But Deirdre and Dr. Giles have really helped me." I still hadn't told him about Grandpa Homer dropping in. His reaction to Dr. Giles' techniques had been discouraging enough.

"I'm really glad you're better. So glad," he said, taking my hand. "But how do you know these . . . people had anything to do with it? How do you know they're not just taking your money and saying they helped you? Maybe you did it all on your own."

"If you would come and meet them, maybe you'd know why I think they helped me."

"Rob, you're right. I'm not very enthusiastic about the . . . the psychic energy healing thing. You know, these people could be charlatans. It might be dangerous. Have you thought of that?"

"I'm not exactly a babe in the woods here. I listened to court cases for over twenty years. I can tell when something's off. And I can tell when something resonates with me. What I'm finding out . . . it, it feels like truth to me. Like I'm finally on the right track."

He shook his head as if he was denying what I was saying. I don't think he knew he was doing it. "I thought it was just for fun. I thought you'd read a few books, make a few friends, and move on. But it's like you're obsessed."

I tried to see it from his side. He was right. I was obsessed—I'd become a spiritual seeker. I was never one to go half measures.

I looked at Aaron. He made it a point to go back to reading his magazine with a disapproving sigh.

"Don't worry," I said. "I'm okay."

Without taking his eyes from the magazine, he asked, "So you coming to the race?"

"Only if I get done in time." I didn't like the stubbornness I heard in my voice.

I started up the car and pulled out of the garage. With gravel spitting out from under my tires, I headed down our long driveway. I didn't want to feel irritated and frustrated . . . but I did.

Even though I knew I'd be late for the author signing, I pulled off the main road and parked in a turnout. Turning off the ignition, I closed my eyes, leaned my head back against the headrest, and let the anger roll off me.

Damn it, I want to share these things with him, not fight about them, I thought.

The previous conversation might not seem like a fight, but it was for us. We didn't like arguing and had rarely left a disagreement hanging unresolved in our whole twenty-two-year marriage. But the past six months, subtle confrontations like that were becoming more frequent. And it was always the same argument. Aaron strongly disapproved of what I was now investigating.

Aaron and I shared similar religious backgrounds. We even went to the same Catholic school as children. We saw each other every Sunday at church. Now our belief systems were diverging. It wasn't that either of us had ever been very devout Catholics. Both of us had stopped going to Sunday services when our lives got so busy. Then when Colin was in second grade we had to decide if we wanted him to take his first communion. Would we raise our child Catholic even though we were hardly practicing that religion? We decided to go ahead; it was our heritage after all. Maybe it was this very apathy to the spiritual side of life that was now the real issue.

I was no longer apathetic. It was like I could hear the singing of my soul calling me onward. I had no doubt I was on a path intended for me from birth, and I was *flying* down that path. I wanted someone to share these beautiful discoveries with, someone to fly down this spiritual path with me.

Aaron wasn't flying down the path. He was holding me back.

The reason that "Huh???" bothered me so much was it was a repeated reminder of the deep gulf opening between us. I tried to talk to him about my impassioned spiritual discoveries, but he would shoot them down as nonsense every time. I found myself defending my new-found beliefs, arguing with Aaron over every new idea. There was no point in that. Besides, I felt like my new discoveries were delicate seedlings I needed to nourish. Why expose them to someone's stomping?

So, eventually, I kept quiet.

But that didn't feel authentic.

And I had an irresistible desire to be authentic. I wanted to be up front about my truth and be taken seriously.

Aaron and I were gradually spending less free time together. Since high school, we'd been inseparable. Now we were going our separate ways on the weekends. I passionately attended my classes and workshops. He pursued his love of aviation and motorcycle racing without me. In the evenings we would eat in silence in the kitchen, then sit in silence in the family room with Aaron watching racing and me reading a book about my latest spiritual passion. We were practically living separate lives already.

The disagreement we just had might have seemed mild to some people, but I could feel the love we shared diminish a tiny bit with each unresolved argument. It was so painful. What we valued most was important to both of us. It wasn't Aaron's fault he wanted to keep spirituality comfortably in the background of our lives—as it always had been up to now. It wasn't my fault it was becoming the most important thing in my life.

His belittlement of the new ideas I was exploring had at first made me feel vaguely embarrassed, as if I should be ashamed to be exploring ideas that were . . . well, perhaps unorthodox. Then I felt disappointed he wasn't more encouraging, at least glad *I* was excited and enlivened by it. As the weeks went by, disappointment was followed by feeling annoyed, frustrated, and finally angry. Lately, anger had been sliding into depression, the depression of being trapped in an environment of disapproval and rejection.

"If we stay together, we're going to end up eventually hating each other."

I realized I had actually said that out loud. It hung in the air like a curse.

I leaned my forehead against the steering wheel and fervently prayed, "Please, God, don't let that happen. Please help me know what to do."

But intuitively I'd known for the past six months what to do, and I was strongly resisting it. Initially I couldn't even imagine it. I couldn't bring myself to even think the word. But it kept looming in the background of my mind . . . *divorce.*

With sadness lodged under my breastbone, I covered my eyes with my arms and cried. Then I sat up.

No. No way.

Ignoring the tiny voice inside me—the voice that had brought out that terrible word—I angrily wiped my tears away. "We've got to find a way to stay together," I affirmed. I resolved to try harder to make this work with Aaron. I would ignore my feelings of unhappiness and mounting frustration. So what if I couldn't share my passion for spiritual exploration? I was going to squelch that little voice inside of me urging me to leave. I would make this work with Aaron. After all, he was a devoted father and a helluva good guy and I knew I was blessed to be with him. I started up the car, took a U-turn, and drove back home.

I could sit through another boat race.

9
"I AM NOT A TEACHER!"

In the late spring of 2000, I was once again on my way to the spiritual bookstore in our town. This weekend they were sponsoring a "psychic fair." You could sign up for a fifteen-minute session from talented psychics who came in from all over the area. Some of my meditation group members said it was a high point of their year. I wasn't exactly sure what made a psychic talented, but it was intriguing.

On my way there, I felt vaguely guilty. I had told Aaron I was going to a book fair, leaving off the psychic part. *I'll stop in and look around,* I told myself. *If I get a bad feeling, I'll just leave.*

When I got there, the place was packed. Watching the excitement of the people waiting to be called for their psychic reading raised my curiosity. It looked like fun, so I decided to give it a whirl.

I located the counter where people were signing up. A young girl with tortoiseshell glasses was sitting at the counter reading. "Can I get in to see someone . . . a . . . uh . . . psychic?" I had a hard time spitting out the word.

"The only one who is available right away is Joy," she said, nodding toward a curly redhead with a quiet demeanor, sitting patiently behind her table with an empty chair across from her. "If you want someone else, you'll have to wait a bit."

I made my way through the packed room and sat across from Joy, who gave me a shy smile.

"I've never done this before. What do I do?" I asked. My voice came out as a blend of apprehension and excitement.

"Is there anything in particular you'd like to know?" Joy asked.

"Not really," I replied. "I was just wanting to try something new. Guess I got caught up in all the excitement."

"Okay. Sit quietly for a minute and I'll see what impressions I get."

With her eyes closed, Joy leaned back in her chair with her hands lying palms up in her lap. Although it was only a few minutes, in my state of anticipation it seemed like an hour before Joy opened her eyes and smiled at me. "Well, I'm getting very strongly you're going to be a teacher."

"A teacher?" I tried not to let her hear my disappointment. *A teacher? Man, is she ever way off base. Never in a million years.*

"That's what I'm getting. You're going to be a teacher." Joy shrugged her shoulders.

I abruptly stood up and extended my hand. "Thanks," I said. I didn't need to hear any more from this woman. Obviously she didn't know what the heck she was talking about. *A teacher! No wonder there isn't any wait for her table.*

Normally I would have walked away and been done with my little psychic experiment. But a little voice inside me said, *Don't leave yet. Try again.* Oh well, I'd come all this way. Why not?

Before I knew it, I found myself back up at the front counter where the gal was scheduling the psychics.

"Who's got the longest line?" I asked.

She grinned showing her dimples. "Martha," she said. "But she's not available for over an hour."

Although I couldn't explain it, I felt this quiet urge to wait for Martha. I was surprised to hear myself say, "Okay. Put me down for Martha."

I browsed through the bookstore and grabbed a book on

mindfulness. With a cup of peppermint tea, I settled into a well-worn gingham chair in the children's section and waited for my appointment.

When my name was called more than an hour later, I walked up to Martha's table. Although Martha had been busy all morning with an endless line, she seemed full of energy. When I had first thought about coming to this event, I think a large part of me expected the psychics to be hanging out in tents in the field behind the store, hovering over a crystal ball, shrouded in smoky layers of incense with their head wrapped in a sequined scarf.

Martha was not that type of psychic. Dressed in her stylish beige jacket and blue blouse with her blond hair in a modern shoulder-length cut, Martha looked like a typical professional woman you might encounter anywhere.

"How can I help you today?" Martha gently clasped her hands and placed them on the table.

"I don't know. I just got this sense I needed to talk to you."

"Well, let's see," Martha answered in a confident voice. She lowered her eyes and sat quietly for a few minutes. I sat motionless across from her, pretending to be observing open-mindedly. Really, there was full-blown judging going on from my side of the table. *She seems nice enough but . . . is this woman for real or a quack?*

Finally Martha took a deep breath and looked up at me. "Well, aren't you the lucky one, three sweet sisters and two awesome brothers. And such loving, devoted parents!"

"How in the world did you know—" I started to say, but cut myself off. She was a psychic. *How did you know?* didn't apply. Still, I was mystified. I had never met this woman before. We had no mutual acquaintances as far as I knew.

"Boy, you've had some health challenges." Martha shook her head. "But it looks like your liver is doing better. How's your memory coming along?" she nonchalantly asked.

Dumbfounded, I sat there in shock. I couldn't move, let alone respond. Thoughts were racing through my head, *What the hell! How does she . . . this is like what happened with Deirdre and my dead Grandpa Homer. How in the world do these people know these things?*

I finally found my voice. "My memory sucks. I can't remember squat. That's why I can't do my job as a court stenographer anymore. It's . . ." I suddenly found myself tearing up. "I . . . um . . . really loved my job . . ." My voice was cracking.

Martha leaned forward, looking compassionately into my face, and handed me a tissue. Something about her kindness set me off, and all the struggles around my work life came gushing out. "I'm volunteering at a veterinary clinic, because I want to help animals heal someday. I love animals so much, I think it's a job I could really enjoy. But I have to keep notes on the simplest things—look. Look at this," I said, pulling my tiny spiral notebook out of my pocket. I opened it and showed it to Martha. She studiously looked at the page that had "Clean a Kennel" scrawled at the top. It listed step-by-detailed-step what I was to do to clean and sterilize a dirty dog kennel. "I've always been such an upbeat person, a model employee, but the staff treat me like an idiot. And they don't even know the half of it. I keep my notebook and my memory problems a secret. I used to be so respected. Attorneys and judges used to ask me for my opinion. Now no one wants to hear a word I say. It's really hard to stay upbeat when you're cleaning kennels for . . . for . . . f-f-free." To my mortification, I started crying so hard I couldn't say any more.

Martha had been patiently listening through all this. Now she handed me another tissue.

"I'm sorry, I don't normally cry like this." I blew my nose and tried to continue. "Have I gone over my fifteen minutes?"

"Don't worry about that," Martha said. "Take your time."

After a long pause, I pulled myself together enough to quietly confess, shaking my head, "I don't know what I'm gonna do for a job now."

"Just take a deep breath," Martha suggested.

After a few deep breaths, I felt a little calmer and started to regain my composure.

We both sat in silence for a few minutes. Martha lowered her gaze and appeared to be listening to a silent conversation at the table I wasn't privy to.

"It's been a rocky road for you, but things will be better from here. Eventually I don't think you will be missing your former career at all. I see that you *will* be working to heal animals. I see you enjoying your work tremendously."

"Really?" I knew it all might be phony. I knew she might just be saying that to encourage me, but for some reason, I felt tremendously reassured.

"And I see something else," Martha continued. "I see you standing in front of a group of people talking to them, and they're totally fascinated by what you're saying. I see you being a teacher."

"I'm not a teacher!" *What is up with this teacher thing?! It's crazy.*

Martha gave me a knowing smile. "I just know that's what I'm getting."

We spoke another ten minutes. Other than the teacher bit, I thought Martha was uncannily accurate. And I got some messages that day that lifted my spirits and gave me courage: "You are right where you need to be. You're on track with your soul's journey. Keep following your heart and you are going to love where you end up."

10
REGARDING SOUL MATES

I stood in my doorway and watched my sixteen-year-old son hop on his bike and take off for his dad's house. I looked at the sky and wondered if he would get home before the rain started. It had been fair earlier, but now the clouds were gathering fast, thick, and black as they frequently were in March.

As I watched my son pedal away, I thought again what a smart, kind, mature, good, responsible, athletic, loving, fun guy he was. Not that I'm prejudiced.

I was so lucky he had weathered the divorce with such grace.

Despite my best efforts to keep my marriage together, it hadn't gotten any better. It had gotten worse.

There were other problems that contributed, but the conflict in our belief systems was primary. Aaron's disapproval of—and my enthusiasm for—my new spiritual pursuits pulled us further and further apart, just as I had feared they would. Listening to my heart, my spiritual studies had been transformational. Although they didn't resonate with Aaron, they made perfect sense to me. They answered my inner questions and brought deep peace to my soul. I was discovering who I really was and how I fit into the world. The bell had been rung. I couldn't unlearn what had awakened me to a greater consciousness about my existence as an evolving soul. The conflict between us grew unbearable.

Yet I spent many a sleepless night wrestling with the impossibility of leaving my husband. Round and round I went:

How can I leave my best friend? Aaron lovingly nursed me through two near brushes with death. How could I be so ungrateful as to leave him now?

How could I break up our family? No more family holidays together, no more getting up Christmas morning to unwrap presents or sharing breakfast or sitting around the table at night, listening to how each other's day had gone.

Will Colin ever forgive me for hurting his father so terribly?

My parents and Aaron love each other so much. I love his parents so much. Will dearest Tillie, Aaron's mother, ever speak to me again?

We're Catholics; divorce is unthinkable—a terrible stigma. We will never be able to get married again in the church. If either of us remarries, we'll be living in sin. My parents will think they raised me wrong.

How in the world will I support myself? I can't work as a highly paid court stenographer anymore. What on Earth will I do to survive?

I still loved Aaron. I knew in my heart I always would. He had been the love of my life since high school. But something inside me wouldn't quit telling me that if I didn't leave, the loss of my true self would smother out the love we had between us. If I waited too long, it wouldn't be a choice; it would be a necessity. And the resentment would turn to a hatred that would kill any chance of us honoring what we had had together and eventually returning to friendship. The lifelong friendship we deserved to have with each other.

Leaving Aaron was the hardest thing I had ever done in my life.

I didn't know if I had the strength to leave the man I loved, my best friend. So I prayed, over and over, *Please guide all of us through this with love and forgiveness.*

I was placing a lot of trust in the inner voice that told me everything would work out all right. One part of me was terrified. Another part was rock solid sure this is what I needed to do.

Divine Love came through.

Aaron and I divorced in December of 2000 and it was completely amicable. We used a single attorney to draw up the papers. There was no conflict, bitterness, or haggling. Although we were both in pain over dissolving our marriage, we remained friends. True, here it was the following March and we weren't seeing much of each other at the moment. But I had faith that after we both had done some healing, we'd be meeting together at family gatherings again with heartfelt love.

Now I tossed some wood in my wood-burning stove and got a good fire crackling. Sure enough, here came the rain. It ran down the picture windows of my living room in great, soggy beads. I sat down in my favorite chair and Checkers jumped up on my lap and rested his head on my arm. "You're such a sweet dog," I said and kissed the top of his head.

Spirit had come through for me in so many ways. It couldn't have been coincidence that at the perfect time I had found this beautiful house to live in only a few miles from our old house where Aaron and Colin were still living.

And . . . the seller had been willing to reduce the price so I could afford to buy it.

And . . . it had a beautifully landscaped yard complete with a graceful white gazebo.

And . . . the yard sloped down to my neighbors' horse pastures, where I could watch the horses graze.

And . . . I had found a much better position at a veterinary office with a wonderful boss, where they actually were going to pay me to be a veterinary assistant.

This was the first time I experienced what happens when you follow the urgings of your soul. The way opens. Things fall into place.

I was still expanding my spiritual landscape—reading, listening, attending classes. In addition, I had started going to gatherings held by a woman named Karyn, who channeled Divine Mother. It was at the urging of Dr. Giles that I had started to attend these sessions. She told me they were transformational, and they were. Again my expectations of how a spiritual counselor should look—who they should be in their ordinary life—were reversed. Karyn called herself a seer and a channel for spirits on the other side, but she was also an adoring mother with small children. The house where we met might have scrawled children's drawings pinned up on the walls and Karyn might be wearing a sweatshirt decorated with little duckies on it for Easter. She was a large-hearted deep-voiced dark-haired mom with an honest face and an enormous embrace. The teachings of Divine Mother that she channeled were remaking me to my core.

I'd like to say that all this gave me an undying faith. I'd like to say that I was happy and that I now felt completely at peace and supported by Divine Love all the time.

I'm sorry to disappoint. Nothing could have been further from the truth. Most of the time I felt totally lost.

I wasn't used to being out in the world on my own. I had been in a relationship, a single relationship, since high school. I had been living in a house filled with family. Now all that was gone.

On this dark and rainy March day, with Colin riding off and the early spring evening coming on, my mind started on its old round of worries again. I stroked and stroked Checkers' ear, and he stirred restlessly.

Everywhere I turned my mind, there was nothing but uncertainty.

I had searched and searched my soul for what my new career should be. I had finally settled on becoming an alternative healer for animals. I had been healed with alternative means; I wanted to provide that to animals. I didn't know of any alternative animal healers nearby, so I decided to see what Western medicine was doing for animals and how that might complement my future healing practice. I sought out a conventional veterinarian for whom I could work. But while my health continued to improve, I wasn't healthy enough to work or study full time yet. Would I ever be?

I had only recently started my new job at Dr. Hamilton's veterinary clinic. Would she find out I had memory impairment, that I had to write down every detail? If she found out, would she fire me?

What I was earning wasn't nearly enough to live on by myself. I was living on savings and my settlement from the divorce. How long would that last? Not forever, that was sure. Should I move, find a cheaper place? But what about Colin? I needed to stay close to him.

On and on my mind ran without getting anywhere, the hamster on the wheel. I didn't know how to make it stop. I didn't know that nighttime was not the best time to hash over your worries, searching for solutions. Frequently, tormenting thoughts would tumble over one another all night long—my old friend, insomnia, was back. And that made me afraid I would exhaust myself and the hepatitis C would take over my body again.

On good days, I would remember to read something inspiring. Perhaps, to focus on my breath for a few minutes and maybe—just maybe—I would be able to quiet my mind for that time.

Slowly, slowly, Spirit was teaching me how to live with uncertainty. How to hand it over. How to stay open to the movement of Spirit in its own time. Divine Love is constantly arranging and rearranging the pieces to fall into place perfectly at the right time. The *how* and the *when*—that is what we have to hand over.

Meanwhile, I was lonely. There had been a lot of evenings like this one. My dog, Checkers, and my cat, Scooter, were wonderful animal companions, but I missed the chatter and noises of a family in the house.

Martha, the woman I had met at the psychic fair a year ago, had become a good friend. On evenings like this I consoled myself by remembering something she had recently told me: A new man would be coming into my life soon. My soul mate.

"Really? What's he like?"

"I can see him quite clearly. He's very good looking, about six-foot, two-inches. He looks good in jeans. I see him working with horses. Very distinguished, confident in his own skin . . . Intelligent—very intelligent. And kind. He has the most beautiful, kind eyes. I can see him sitting in front of a fireplace in a house with high vaulted ceilings and cedar beams. He's looking into the fire and he's thinking of you. He doesn't know it's you yet, but he's dreaming of his own soul mate coming into his life."

On dark, rainy evenings like this, when all the uncertainties of my life would crowd in on me, I would picture that. I would picture this man who was my soul mate sitting in front of his fireplace in his living room with the high-beamed ceiling, reading or gazing at the fire just as I was doing now. Any day now he would come walking into my life.

Of course, when he did come, my soul mate did not walk into my life. He rolled in to it . . . in a wheelchair. That was one little detail Martha inadvertently left out.

11

A QUIET MAN

Martha's farm-style yard was filled with people on the Fourth of July, and all of them were fascinating. Especially the man in front of me, Jason—handsome, tall, and the author of a book on animal healing. If I could read the signals (and let's face it, at this age I had been doing that a long time), he was interested in me. He was asking me if I'd like to ride with him while he ran out to buy more ice. I sure would.

It was the summer of 2001, a year and a half after I had left my home and my marriage. I was continuing to improve physically and I was able to work several hours a day at Dr. Hamilton's veterinary clinic. I was moving ahead with my plans to create a new career working with animals and still exploring the new world of spirituality that had opened up for me.

You could write a *Who's Who* volume based on the people who were at the party that day. When Martha had invited me, my secret reaction was, *Ohhh! I can't believe I get to be invited to this party!* Martha knew everybody I wanted to meet. There were at least fifty or sixty people coming and going, open-house style. Alternative medicine healers, authors, spiritual teachers, animal communicators . . . people who made me gulp when they were pointed out. *Really? That's so and so?* With my interest in alternative medicine for animals, this seemed like a once-in-a-lifetime event. I was pretty pumped.

After arriving at the party and grabbing a plate, I drifted from group to group, looking for interesting discussions. People had spilled out from the open doors of Martha's three-bedroom rambler and scattered into the yard. The house was surrounded by pastures with horses and cows peacefully grazing. Everywhere were little impromptu circles of outdoor chairs filled with people in animated conversation between bites of picnic food. It looked like a typical Fourth of July cookout—jeans, shorts and sandals, laughter and heaped plates—but the snatches of conversation made it clear it was anything but typical.

". . . What I love about using the points for acupressure is the owner can use them on the pet at home . . ."

". . . She's moving to Hawaii to be closer to the dolphins there, but I think she'll be coming back twice a year to still run the orca excursions . . ."

". . . He's been using the heart chakra bowl during the meditations and the light has been phenomenal . . ."

As I circulated I heard talk of a particular energy healer who hadn't arrived yet, but was expected any minute. He had clinics in California, and stories about miraculous healings that had happened with him were being passed around with the drink refills. Martha and her husband-to-be, Parker, were opening a big alternative-medicine clinic, and several of the people there that day were considering becoming a part of it. Parker explained to me they were hoping this particularly gifted energy healer—Dr. Gary Holz—would be an anchor store, like a Nordstrom or a Macy's, for the new clinic.

I almost missed Gary's arrival by departing on my ice run. But Jason left me to grab his car keys and was delayed by other fascinating guests on the way. By the time he came back, *I* was in yet another non-stoppable conversation. I saw Jason waiting off to the side, but I just couldn't break off the talk. Jason could see how enthralled I was and he didn't want to interrupt, so he left without me.

What would have happened to my life if I hadn't met Gary that day? What would have happened if I'd taken off with Jason and never returned to the party? Or come back after Gary left? When I look back, I can see the little twists of timing that were Divine Love looking out for me, the oh-so-subtle pushes in the right direction. But that day I hadn't a clue where I was headed.

When Gary arrived, there was quite a stir. I didn't really pay attention to the van that had pulled in until people rushed toward it. I only peripherally noted the dignified man, with salt-and-pepper hair and beard, roll down the van's ramp in a wheelchair. I caught a glimpse of a slim, strong man, well dressed, wearing jeans and a nice shirt. His demeanor was unassuming, quiet, and reserved. Four or five people stepped up to help him, get him food, introduce themselves. *So this was who everybody had been waiting for. Hmmm.* He was quickly surrounded and I continued my discussion.

The party bubbled on. Eventually, I wanted to join a conversation that was taking place in a group of chairs circled together beside Martha's faded red barn. The only empty seat was next to Gary's wheelchair. I moved to take it and someone standing nearby introduced us. He took my hand. His eyes locked on my face and his expression seemed to freeze for a moment.

I didn't find out until years later what happened to Gary in that few seconds during which we shook hands.

As he extended his hand, my face changed before his eyes, becoming the face of someone else. It was as if another woman's face became superimposed over mine. And he recognized this woman—he knew this was the face of someone he had known and dearly loved in a previous life. Nothing like this had ever happened to him before.

Then my face shifted again. Another face was imposed over mine, and it was yet another love from another lifetime.

The queue continued. One face after another, at least a dozen times.

Gary was completely nonplussed. From my open expectant expression he could tell I was not sharing in this display of our past-life relationships. I was smiling and shaking hands with no sign of recognition at all.

"Nice to meet you, Gary."

Gary had no idea what to say. In this lifetime, we had never met, and yet this was a soul he had known—and dearly loved—many times before. It was obvious to him that *to me* this was nothing more than a very casual meeting between two strangers at a party of a mutual acquaintance. What do you say to someone in a situation like that? Evidently, not much.

"Hi," he said.

We sat side by side in comfortable silence. I listened to the conversations in the circle, eventually joining in.

The afternoon was waning and in typical Northwest fashion the July day had become chilly. One of Gary's admirers came over and asked him if he would like a blanket. Before they could return with it, he rolled off to his van, maybe to take a moment to regroup after his odd experience while meeting me. Gary's friend came back with the blanket. I was wearing shorts and sandals and felt like I was two degrees Fahrenheit away from hypothermia, so I graciously offered to hold the blanket and give it to Gary when he returned.

When Gary returned, I said, "Here's your blanket. I was warming it up for you."

"Thank you," he said, taking the blanket and looking away quickly.

This was the man who would change my life forever, and at our first meeting he spoke three words to me: "Hi" and "Thank you."

We parted company and I hadn't felt a thing. No Fourth of July fireworks going off, no chills running up and down my spine, no flashing lights spelling, *Robbie! This is the one!* in my head. The Earth didn't move, it didn't even quiver.

But from that moment forward I was headed into an unimaginable adventure. Sometimes you can put your foot on a new, life-shattering path and not even know it.

12

A JOB OFFER

After his experience at the Fourth of July picnic, Gary knew I was the one. There was a little problem, however: *I* didn't know it. How was he going to help me see we were destined to be together without appearing to be a crazed stalker?

For my part, I didn't give the quiet man in a wheelchair another thought until two weeks later when I got a call from Martha. Gary had asked her to call me. He wasn't going to be joining Martha and Parker in their clinic, but he was opening a solo practice not too far from me. He had expressed an interest in having me come to work for him when he opened his clinic in a few months.

At the time, I was happy in my job as a veterinary assistant for Dr. Hamilton. I was learning a lot about the techniques of Western veterinary medicine, and I loved Dr. Hamilton herself. She was caring and energetic. I could tell she loved her patients—the animals. In spite of my recovering state and occasional lapses in memory, she gave me a wide range of duties. She treated me with respect. I felt challenged and valued. Why should I leave?

I thanked Martha for passing on the offer and asked her to tell Gary, "Thank you, but I'm not interested at this time."

I didn't know how quietly determined Gary could be.

A week later, he called me himself. He really wanted to work with me. He could tell I loved animals and much of his work was with animals, especially horses, in his California practice. Although I was flattered, I wasn't convinced it was for me.

Even though Martha had told me that the man coming into my life was working with horses, it never occurred to me it could be Gary. I was completely blind to the possibility.

Gary didn't give up. He sent me an e-mail. And Martha mentioned it again. And it came up in conversation with another friend. Gary called once or twice more about it. I was stalwart. "Sorry, I'm really happy working where I am."

Then Gunner came in with a broken back, and I made that call to Gary. After I had visited his new clinic several times with Gunner, and witnessed Gunner's healing, Gary made me an offer I couldn't refuse: "Come to work for me and I'll teach you how I heal animals."

I thought of Gunner. I thought of Gary saying, "I'll be right there." Something about that phrase reverberated in me and gave me a warm glow. I thought of the excitement I had felt seeing that miraculous healing.

I said okay.

But I didn't leave Dr. Hamilton's office right away. Gary's clinic wasn't scheduled to open for another two months, and there were details about the job I wanted to iron out. I wanted to make sure I could do the work Gary would be expecting of me. My health had improved tremendously. To outside eyes I was normal, energetic even, but I still needed thirteen to fourteen hours of sleep a day, which included a midday nap. If I overdid it on the exercise or work, it could bring on a headache that sent me back to bed for a day or more.

And there was another complication. I could usually tell if someone was romantically interested in me, and I knew Gary was courting me. Because I had agreed to work with Gary, I had no intention of starting a romantic relationship with him. I wasn't going to leave the job I loved with Dr. Hamilton only to complicate my new prospects with an office romance.

I won't say his wheelchair made no difference to me at all. Of course it did. But in spite of that I found Gary to be a very attractive man. Intelligent and powerful in a way I had never known before. Over the next few months, as he got his new practice opened and running, he would call me in the evenings and we'd talk about our days. He was so shy during our calls that I had trouble hearing half of what he said. I found that contrast—shy and powerful—intriguing.

One day in the early fall, he called and asked me to go to lunch with him. I thought we were going to make plans for my new job. Looking back, I realize he thought it was a date.

I met him at a nice restaurant in a location midway between his new clinic and where I was still working with Dr. Hamilton. He was already seated at the table when I arrived.

"Hi, I hope I'm not late."

"No . . . no."

"Oh, good."

A few seconds of quiet. I took a breath, but no idea for a conversational opener came out.

Now I'm really comfortable with talking. I can make a conversation with an abalone clinging to its rock. But I will tell you, this was the most uncomfortable lunch I have ever had. Gary was so quiet, so soft-spoken during this lunch, I couldn't hear most of what he said. It took me several tries to hear his answers to every one of my questions. After we had talked—halting and stuttering and floundering—regarding when I would start work, and what my work schedule would be, we still had the rest of an hour to get through. It went something like this:

"So, I know you teach classes and workshops. Are you teaching energy healing?"

"I . . . mhmsspf . . . rspmsifflepumf."

"I'm sorry. I didn't get that." I lean in and cock an ear.

"Well . . ." He draws back slightly, so I lean forward even more, straining to hear. "Kuhpmflslpk . . . iscramnfnt."

"So sorry, could you say that last part again?" I lean in more, trying not to look like I'm doing it.

"Bliklmnt . . . frmantrof . . . spishm."

"Ah, and will I be mostly watching then? To learn, I mean. Or were you thinking I would meet with you for instruction?"

"You . . . pflmansus mimush rotoff nofer."

"Uh-huh. Do you treat a lot of animals?"

The dear man. He was so intimidated by the challenge of winning me over he could not raise his voice. I had no clue what was wrong. He couldn't possibly be so shy with everyone. The man had taught workshops on Aboriginal healing all up and down the coast for goodness sake. What was the matter with him?

If three tries didn't do it, I gave up and tried another conversation starter. In any social circle, a lunch like that is considered damn hard work. At the end of the entrée, I was so frustrated that I literally couldn't wait to get out of there.

If I can only catch the waitress's eye. *No, no. I never eat dessert* (a total lie). *No coffee thanks, I gotta get back to work, you know.*

I still feel bad about what happened next. I don't know what came over me. Mom, I would just like to say you raised me better than this, but I was so uncomfortable, escape was my only thought.

At this restaurant you paid at a glass-fronted counter near the entrance. Gary was going to pay for lunch and I thanked him. We walked up to the front and instead of waiting with him for the hostess to arrive and then walking out with him, I just said, "Well, 'bye," and left him at the counter!

This is a man in a wheelchair. I didn't know at the time how challenging it was for him to get in and out of his van. It was a steep uphill roll. I could have seen him out, offered to help, but no. I was so anxious to get away from this horrible lunch, I just thanked him and bolted out of there.

A couple days later, I saw Martha.

She said, "I hear you and Gary had a nice lunch together."

"What?!"

"He said it went *really* well."

"You gotta be kidding me!"

He thought that went really well? At that point, I had no doubts. No way did I want to get involved with someone so socially inept. No way did I want to get involved with my future boss. No way did I want to get involved with a paraplegic.

But all that was to change—like the flipping of a light switch—because of what he was about to do for my sister, who was going blind.

13

ANN

My sister Ann had a rare eye disease called uveitis, an inflammation of both irises that was slowly destroying her vision. She was looking out at the world through a white, blurry haze. All that remained of her sight was some peripheral vision in her left eye. She was a forty-three-year-old happily married mother still living in our home state of Illinois, and she would soon be completely blind.

Because the disease was so rare, there was little or no research being done on it at that time, and local doctors had done all they could for her. Her situation was alarmingly similar to how I had been left with my hepatitis C. There was no known cure in 2001.

From my distance in the Northwest, I had kept track of her search for a cure down every avenue. She had tried every possibility she could dig up and spent all their savings traveling to different places where someone offered a possible cure, only to experience no improvement and a steady progress of the blindness. It was unbearably sad.

Throughout the fall and into the winter of 2001, Gary and I continued with our phone conversations several times a week. In one of our phone calls, I described Ann's situation.

He suggested she should come see him.

In spite of having seen the healing of Gunner and having heard other stories of Gary's healing abilities, I might not have gotten behind the idea if I had relied on my rational mind. But when Gary suggested it, from somewhere deep inside came a strong conviction: *Gary can help Ann. We should bring her out here.*

My logic and fears immediately jumped in. What if Gary couldn't help her? What if she spent all that money to come out here and only had her hopes dashed? Would her husband agree? What of the children? If all she could afford was a short visit, would Gary still be able to help? The thoughts cascaded around in my mind. But during the times I was most peaceful, during my meditation time or when I was enjoying a beautiful sunset, the thought returned: *Gary can help Ann. You should bring her out.* It felt like the advice was coming from my heart and I decided to act on it. I threw myself into the project.

It was with total trust in me—and a thin thread of hope—that Ann flew from Illinois to have Gary treat her "incurable" uveitis. The earliest we could arrange the trip was for late January. She was accompanied by one of my other sisters (in fact, Ann's twin sister, Melinda). Ann and Melinda were to stay with me and we would travel to Gary's house for treatments, which was located outside a midsized town named Keyserville sixty miles away.

My sisters were only able to be here for five days. We had five days to try to accomplish a miraculous cure.

Gary's house was a beautiful place surrounded by majestic evergreens on a steep hill above Lake Samantha. The entire house, first and second stories, had been designed to take advantage of the expansive view. The living room where Ann received her treatments had floor-to-ceiling windows that looked out past a deck to the serene lake spread far below.

Gary saw Ann every day. The treatments were surprisingly brief. Gary would work on Ann by placing his left hand at the back of her neck for a few minutes, leave her resting on one of his butter-soft leather couches for twenty to thirty minutes, and return after that to place his hand on the back of her neck a second time. Then we would return home.

I didn't understand what Gary was doing. He had vaguely explained to me he was using his mind and touch as a channel for a healing energy. Although Gary had penned his book about his experiences with the Aboriginals, it was not published yet and I had never read it. Nor had I had the chance to attend one of his workshops on Aboriginal healing. So I had no clue what was going on beyond what I saw with my physical eyes.

One morning during Ann's five-day stay, we girls woke up to . . . snow. Only a Seattleite can understand the terror that word can strike in the breast of someone who lives in this area. When it snows in the Seattle area, it's a totally different matter than when it snows in the Midwest or Maine. We are not physically set up for snow. The land is hilly. Out in the sticks where we lived, no snowplows, salt, or sand spreaders were going to show up—forget it. That snow was gonna stay right where it was until it melted. But the real problem when it snows in our area is that the inhabitants seem to go crazy, driving with a fantastical lack of judgment only the truly panicked can exhibit. Which means that when it snows in Seattle—the city stops. Ninety percent of the population hunkers down for the duration (usually only a few days) and waits for the return of warmer temperatures and blessed rain to wash all that white stuff away.

Ann had only five days to get her treatments and now we might not be able to get there for them. Gary's house was at the top of a long, steep, winding driveway that would have been considered completely impassable by Northwest natives when covered with snow. Good thing we girls weren't Northwest natives.

My sisters and I were raised in the Midwest. It snows there. Frequently. Added to that, we all had the tenacious can-do attitude to match the situation. If Ann needed further treatments in her remaining days, we'd find a way to somehow get her to Gary. So we loaded up my Honda station wagon with emergency supplies, shovels in case we slid into a bank, and cat litter and rugs to throw under the tires for added traction if we needed it. Decked out in boots, gloves, scarves, and hats, we set out heavily armed with determination, resourcefulness, and will.

It was a snap. The Seattle natives had stayed home, and we cautiously made our way through the beautiful snow-blanketed countryside. Gary had called earlier that morning to warn us about his driveway, but we managed it with only a little bit of slipping.

Three heavily clad women with smiles, hats, snow-covered boots and gloves, and a great deal of enthusiasm burst into his home. "We made it!" I cried out to him.

Usually, I would perch on the arm of the couch, trying to make socially awkward moments more comfortable (with all Gary's gifts, social skills were not high on the list). But sometimes, while the others were busy, I would wander around the house taking in the beautiful paintings and statues, many of which were gifts from former patients.

During this visit, I stood at the kitchen sink and gazed out the window at the beauty of the evergreens with their massive branches covered in snow. Ann was having her break between healing sessions and Gary was sitting quietly in his wheelchair.

Suddenly, the idea popped into my mind, *Wouldn't you like to marry Gary and live here in this beautiful house?*

My immediate response was an incredulous, *No!* Followed by, *Where the heck did that thought come from?!*

It wasn't until years later I discovered Gary's telepathic abilities. I have no doubt he put that thought in my mind. Somehow, I don't think that was the response he was hoping for.

We continued to go to Gary's house every day for treatments despite the snow.

One night, back at my house, Ann awoke in the dark. A slide show was passing before her eyes. She sat up in bed and watched as little boxes of dark and light images—they looked like photographic negatives—moved from left to right in front of her eyes. She could not interpret any of the images. They looked like nothing she had ever seen before. This continued until she slipped back into sleep. The next day she asked

Gary about it, and he told her in his soft, succinct way, "Your eyes are reprogramming themselves."

On the third evening, Gary took me aside as we were getting ready to leave his house. "I don't want you to tell your sisters, but I think Ann is going to have a breakthrough," he said quietly.

"When?"

"Tomorrow morning."

Although we had seen no improvement in the three days Ann had been receiving treatment from Gary, I went to bed that night nursing hope.

The next morning I awoke to shouts coming from my living room. My heart pounding, I rushed out to see Ann standing there with her twin sister. They were both still in pajamas with their arms flung around each other in front of the big picture window. Ann was looking out the window at my snow-covered yard and the beautiful pastures below.

With tears running down her face, she was crying out, "I can see! I can see!"

Then, all three of us were in tears as we recognized the significance of what was happening. Ann's vision had started to return.

14

A SUDDENNESS OF LOVE

The last day of Ann's treatment with Gary was in his clinic in Benton. I sat in his waiting room with Melinda, contemplating what had happened here—the immensity of it. After she had spent five days getting treatments from Gary, Ann was going to be returning home to the flat farmland of Illinois with much of her vision restored.

Ann had been healed.

But in a way, I was healed too—because after this nothing would ever look the same. My world had expanded yet again.

How many miracles do you have to witness before you really get it? I had been impressed by the healing of Gunner, the dog with the broken back, but somehow this was different. My sister had been mostly blind and now she could see.

The miracle of it pierced through the resistance of my conscious mind. It was as if the pieces of my world rearranged and fell into a new pattern. I knew: *Miracles are possible.* Joyful, unexpected, inexplicable miracles. I knew: *There is a healing and loving power in the universe.* Call it whatever you want to. Call it Divine Love. It's there and it can be accessed. And Gary had been a vehicle for it.

I felt a profound wave of gratitude wash over me. Although he had never said a word, I suddenly realized Gary had healed Ann out of love for me. I don't know how I knew it, but somehow Ann's healing had been inextricably tied to Gary's love for me.

In that moment, I opened myself to the love Gary had for me, and it poured in. The awareness of it filled me to the center of my being. There was so much. Gary loved me so much. What overcame me next was totally unexpected—I fell instantly in love with this compassionate, quiet healer.

Joy flooded my heart and overflowed. Tears flooded my eyes and also overflowed. I reached into my purse on the floor and grabbed a tissue.

Melinda, who had been leafing through a gardening magazine, looked over at me. "You okay?" she asked.

"Yes, I'm fine," I answered, wiping tears with my tissue and reaching for more. For some reason this didn't convince her.

"What's wrong?" Melinda put down her magazine, concern all over her sweet face.

"Nothing's wrong." I smiled to reassure her. "I just realized something."

I didn't want to wait and assess this feeling. I had to act on it and act now. I stood up and tucked my casual top into my jeans. "I'm going to talk to Gary for a second. I'll be right back."

"Okay." Melinda looked puzzled, but she let me go. "I'll go check on Ann and see how she's doing."

"I think she's resting in the back office," I said, pointing to the room at the far end of the hall.

I had seen Gary leave the back room, where he had been treating Ann, and slip into his office a few minutes before. The door was slightly ajar and I knocked softly as I peeked in. "Can I talk to you for a second?" I asked. I could feel a shy smile on my face, but I was helpless to prevent it.

Gary looked up from the patient chart he had been making notes on and a big smile spread across his face. "Of course. Come in." He put his pen down and closed the folder, then skillfully wheeled his chair around the side of his large wooden desk and pushed the levers down on both wheels to safely lock them in place.

I silently closed the door behind me. When I turned to face him, he looked a little surprised.

"Have a seat," he motioned toward the plush black leather chair across from his desk.

"Actually, I'd rather sit here." I pointed to his lap. "That all right with you?"

He sounded almost giddy as he stammered, "Yeah . . . Sssure. Yes!"

I sat on his lap and put my arms around his neck. My face pressed close to his, I looked into his beautiful warm eyes and said, "Thank you for helping my sister."

"You're . . . you're welcome," he said.

The woodsy scent of the cologne he was wearing was intoxicating. It felt new and exciting to be so close to his strong chest, to feel his arms resting gently around me.

"I know you did that for me." I felt immense gratitude welling up in my heart again.

"It was my pleasure," he quietly replied.

I hesitated. The new feelings inside me toward this kind healer were overwhelming. They had only gotten stronger now that I was in his arms. I wasn't sure how to express them, but I decided to plunge ahead and let it out, come what may.

"I don't know what's happened inside me." I smiled as I gazed into his eyes. "But I feel like a switch has been flipped." I took a deep breath and timidly worked my way through the words. "I've fallen in love with you."

His eyes widened in surprise and his mouth opened as if to speak, but nothing came out. After a brief hesitation, he placed his hand behind my head and pulled my face toward his. He kissed me tenderly on the mouth. "I love you," he said softly and kissed me again. It was sweet and gentle and thoroughly delicious.

We slipped into our own private communion, ecstatic with the realization that we loved each other. We continued to kiss and talk about our feelings and kiss again, oblivious to the world around us, for a long time.

Joining my sisters later in the lobby, I felt like we were a couple of teenagers holding hands in front of our friends for the first time.

My sisters greeted us with knowing looks. "There sure was a lot of laughter coming out of that office," Melinda commented.

Gary and I looked at each other. Try as I might, I just couldn't stop grinning.

15

GARY'S TRIP TO AUSTRALIA

Gary's early life contained no clue he would end up being an energy healer. He was a scientist—a pragmatic scientist. The kind who believes if a phenomenon is not repeatable with measurable results, then it is not a fact. And that means it has no bearing on the real world and you ignore it. Black and white.

Holz Industries was the name of the aerospace company Gary founded during his scientific career. The company had contracts with NASA and various foreign governments around the world. Gary held several U.S. patents for instrumentation he had designed. There were also many other inventions he could have patented, but they were classified top secret and, therefore, sequestered. He frequently made presentations to large numbers of other scientists at conferences. He was by anyone's standards a successful physicist.

Then came the diagnosis of multiple sclerosis (MS).

Gary was diagnosed in 1983. By 1985, he was walking with canes. By 1988, he was using a wheelchair. By 1992, he was for the most part confined to the wheelchair. In 1994, the doctors told him he had less than two years to live. He was only forty-three years old and he had less than two years to live.

Shortly after the prediction of his death by his doctors—feeling totally alone and depressed—Gary went to a local jazz bar. It was crowded and he just happened to sit next to a woman who was originally from Australia. She just happened to know of a healer, Ray, who she thought could help Gary. Ray was part of a remote Aboriginal community living in the Outback, but spent part of his time in a city. She just happened to have his number on her. Even more astounding, Gary felt an irresistible urge to call this Aboriginal man and do whatever Ray might suggest.

A week later in September of 1994, this scientist who had devoted his life to provable facts and logic rolled his wheelchair onto a plane bound for Australia. He was headed to an isolated Aboriginal community settlement not on any map. He was headed to the remote desert in the Australian Outback—all based on the terse, almost cryptic, suggestions of an Aboriginal healer named Ray whom Gary had never met in person. No one in his family accompanied him. They didn't want to encourage him. They thought Gary was behaving like a crazy man.

Even before Gary contacted Ray, the Aboriginal village knew Gary was coming. Community members had been notified in their Dreamtime meditations that a white man would be coming to their village and they were directed to teach him their healing techniques. It was time for their ancient knowledge to be shared with the Western world—knowledge that had developed over the course of their at least 60,000-year-old culture, knowledge they had safeguarded from dilution by white culture for centuries.

You cannot imagine what a stretch this was for these people. The twenty-four members of the village were very reluctant to have a white man come into their settlement. First of all, nobody—except for the two healers, Ray and Rose—had ever been exposed to a white person. It is part of this tribe's tradition that you are not to speak to a person who is not "related to you," has not been given a traditional "name" that explains their relationship to you. Aboriginal ideas of relationship are extremely complex and I cannot begin to explain them. Even Rose had to stay in a hut outside the village because she didn't have a traditional "family" relationship with the community.

It was especially challenging for tribal members to go the next step: *Not only are you going to have a white man come and live with you, but you're also going to teach him your healing techniques.* The messages from the Big Guy must have been powerful and insistent for the community to take it on. But they did; through Ray, they invited Gary to come.

A note here for the feminists among us: Sometimes in this book, I will report Aborigines referring to "The Big Guy." This is a traditional translation given to Europeans for the Aboriginal word for Creator/ Great Spirit/Divine Love. I am told that the original word is without gender, but most of the European colonists in the 1700s to 1800s couldn't comprehend that, so the Aborigines chose the most friendly sounding, nonthreatening name they could come up with in English. It is my understanding that the Aborigines use it a little tongue-in-cheek.

The Aboriginal community had spent a couple of months preparing for Gary before he even knew they existed. Rose was a half-Aboriginal, half-white healer who ran a healing clinic for Aboriginal people and could speak English fluently. They arranged for her to come to the village, so she could communicate with him and teach him their healing techniques using language and metaphors a Westerner could understand.

The Aborigines Gary visited taught him our reality is created at a source level—a spiritual level of reality in the Dreamtime—before manifesting in our sensed world. We can't know for sure what happened at the source level during Gary's stay in the village. Gary later believed the community visualized him walking and feeling, visualized his body whole and healthy, without the MS. They were working at the energetic level, repatterning Gary's body and mind in the Dreamtime. And they were working with his guiding angels and guides, whom they could see and communicate with.

Meanwhile, Rose and Ray talked to him at a conscious level about the Aboriginal principles of healing. They helped him understand that body, mind, and spirit are all one connected whole, and that he had to heal the emotional and subconscious components of his MS before he could heal his body.

Before he left the Outback, after only ten days' time with the Aboriginal community, Gary had recovered feeling in parts of his numb body that hadn't had feeling for seven years. After being bound to the wheelchair for two years, he clumsily walked down the airplane aisle on the return flight home.

More importantly, Gary's eyes had been opened to an expansive spiritual reality. The world was no longer a flat black and white—it extended into new colors of possibility in all directions. During his spiritual experiences with the Aborigines, Gary had been instructed to share what he had learned about healing. He wrote the first draft of his book, *Secrets of Aboriginal Healing*, on the flight home.

Gary always believed the Aboriginal community members, and Rose and Ray, had cured him of his MS. Still, he was never completely free of the wheelchair. He told friends he never fully healed the damage the disease had already wrought on his body. The MS was gone, and his physical condition was greatly improved, but his wheelchair remained.

Two years later, in February of 1996, Gary returned to the Aboriginal settlement to say, "You guys didn't finish the job. Let's get me totally healed."

The community answered through Ray, "The rest is up to you, mate. It's between you and the Big Guy."

During Gary's first stay in the village, Ray had introduced Gary to his primary spirit guide, Julie. Westerners might say Julie was Gary's guardian angel. The Aborigines of this community were aware of spirit guides and able to communicate with them. They communicated freely, not only with their own spirit guides but with other people's.

Gary was not proficient in seeing and communicating with spiritual beings—he had never even considered such a thing. To begin communicating with Julie, Ray invited Gary to ask Julie for a physical sensation that would indicate a "yes" answer to a question. Gary felt a faint touch on his right earlobe. Then he asked for the sensation that would indicate a "no," and felt a faint touch on his left earlobe. Ray considered this a crude way to communicate with your spirit guardian but promised Gary that he would eventually grow into conversing with Julie telepathically. Gary's expanding relationship with Julie changed the course of his life forever.

Before Gary left the Outback, he was told he would become a gifted healer back in the Western culture—the idea was completely new to Gary. He was a physicist. *What do you mean a healer?*

16

YES, A HEALER

The first time Gary channeled healing energy was for his housemate after he had arrived back in the states.

Shauna shuffled into the kitchen like a ninety-year-old woman even though she was only in her thirties. Her shagged blond hair hung in her face, her eyes were opened to slits, and her skin hung loose and tinged with gray.

"Shauna, you look terrible," Gary commented.

"Ughh. Migraine. It happens every damn month just before my period. Sometimes coffee helps." The cup made a slight clunk on the counter, and she winced and swallowed as if suppressing a wave of nausea. "I think they're getting worse though." There was no doubt she was in excruciating pain.

Then, a surprising thing happened. Gary had a feeling he could help her, and he acted on that impulse. Gary had Shauna sit in an overstuffed chair in the living room where he could roll his wheelchair behind her. Then, following his intuition, he placed his left hand on the back of her neck.

He felt healing energy pass through him and into Shauna. The energy seemed to have its own intelligence. It knew where to go and what it needed to do. Gary visualized Shauna well, free of her headache.

He watched passively, *seeing* in his mind's eye, as the blood vessels in her head constricted just the right amount to relieve the pressure. He saw it healed.

"Oh, that feels much better," Shauna mumbled. "Thank you." What he was perceiving was actually happening! It seemed perfectly natural. And Gary realized that he had *known* what he was seeing in his mind was actually happening. Seeing the healing in his mind had been part of the healing process.

Gary continued to be a channel for the healing energy for a few minutes more and left Shauna sleeping peacefully in the chair, head resting back, her breathing deep and easy. Color was returning to her cheeks.

Using the techniques Ray had taught him to communicate with Julie, his guiding angel, Gary asked, *Is she all right? Can I leave her this way?* He felt the gentle sensation—a touch on his right earlobe—that meant *Yes.*

Gary gave Shauna a few more sessions of the healing energy. Her headaches not only subsided that week, but they never returned. Premenstrual migraines were never a problem for her again.

I can only guess what changes were happening in Gary's psyche as he transitioned from being a physicist to an energy healer. He must have been on fire with inspiration.

He began by reading everything he could get his hands on about the body and its pathology. When I met him he had an extensive library. He studied neurology and the mechanics of physical healing. He studied everything he could find that discussed how the mind influences the physical processes of the body. He wanted to know exactly how the body healed itself—what physically needed to happen—because he wanted to be able to direct or support that healing process. He also sought out everything he could find about the body/mind/spirit connection and the blueprint of source energy from which a physical body is created.

He had sold his aerospace engineering company, Holz Industries, and during 1994 and 1995, he used the proceeds to return to school and study immunology, obtaining a masters and then a doctoral degree. His particular interest was in psychoneuroimmunology, the interaction of the mind with the neurotransmitters of the body. He knew a degree in immunology would help him integrate the Aboriginal principles with Western scientific knowledge, and make the principles easier to teach to Westerners.

Knowing the significant effect food has on health and healing, he also earned a degree in nutrition.

Gary began healing friends and friends of friends who asked for his help. Then, he started working on their pets and other animals. He found himself working often on horses. (Remember Martha telling me that she saw my future life-partner working with horses?)

When Gary worked on horses, even the temperamental race horses accepted him rolling around them in his wheelchair. They calmly allowed him to reach up and touch various parts of their bodies. They would gingerly step to one side making room for his wheelchair beside them in their stalls, always conscious of where he was, always careful not to hurt him in any way.

As I witnessed during the healing of Gunner, most animals felt the healing energy and peace Gary exuded right away. Even jittery or frightened animals would calm down in Gary's presence.

Gary's healing successes started mounting up and he opened a clinic in California and called it the Holz Healing Center. As his business grew, he opened up another clinic farther north where he worked on weekends, traveling alone between the two clinics in a van that had been specially customized for his wheelchair.

The Aborigines had asked Gary to share their healing principles with the Western world, and he took that assignment to heart. He wrote articles and a regular column for local health journals and he began teaching three-day workshops titled "Aboriginal Healing Techniques." In his workshops Gary taught a five-step healing process derived from his work with Rose. It was the same process he had recorded on the plane back from Australia and that he planned to eventually publish in a book.

One of Gary's greatest beliefs was in the power of a focused mind to affect healing. The mind/body/spirit connection—it was powerful stuff and a relatively new concept for a lot of people in the late '90s. He taught that when the mind was combined with the limitless healing capabilities of Divine Source, astounding things could happen.

After teaching a seminar in Vancouver, Canada, Gary stayed for an extended time here in Washington state. He fell in love with the area. He decided to move his healing practice and his home base to the Northwest. He made friends and bought a house for a soul mate whom he hadn't met yet. That's when he was introduced to a woman named Robbie at a Fourth of July party and realized she was the one.

17

MANY LIVES

It was three months after my sister Ann returned to Illinois no longer blind, and I was still deeply, madly, excruciatingly in love.

I leaned my chin on my hand and gazed out over the waterfront dock lined with white sailboats, their masts swaying gently on the tranquil water, their sails wrapped in bright blue canvas. The sun was shining brightly on the snow-covered mountains across the Sound, but inside the restaurant it was shadowy and the candlelight shimmered over crisp white tablecloths. It could not have been more romantic and my heart was full to the top and overflowing.

"This is beautiful," I said and reached across the table for Gary's hand.

My petite hand was immediately dwarfed as both of his surrounded mine with a tenderness that warmed me through and through. I loved his hands, his healer's hands. I even loved the tufts of soft brown hair peeking out from the cuffs of his dress shirt.

"You look nice tonight," I said. Gary always had a subtle elegance. Tonight he was in a neatly ironed shirt, dress pants, and Italian leather shoes.

He smiled. "So do you, sweetheart. It's a pretty dress." I was wearing a sleeveless black cocktail dress, and I sat and appreciated him appreciating it.

One of the things the Aborigines had returned to Gary was the ability to have a fulfilling sex life, and I was definitely benefiting from their gift.

I have to admit the physical attraction surprised me. I knew that Gary's gentle, kind, and loving nature would always melt my heart, but I found myself incredibly physically attracted to his strong, lean body and his handsome, sculpted face. He had the most beautiful eyes. Sometimes they looked blue and sometimes green, but they were always decorated with soft, gold flecks. Those eyes with the golden flecks could reach out and pull me in until the rest of the world disappeared. On top of that, the brilliance of his mind was alluring and had an aphrodisiacal effect on me. I found myself mesmerized for hours as I listened to him talk in depth about anything and everything. From the mechanics of putting up satellites in deep space to the inner workings of the heart, I couldn't find a topic he didn't know something about. I could listen to him talk endlessly.

"Thanks for taking me to dinner here. This place is one of my favorites."

"I thought you'd like it." Gary smiled back at me.

"How was your day?"

He chuckled. "Not what my lawyer expected."

"What happened?" I asked.

"I met with Todd this morning about incorporating the business in Washington."

"Good." I nodded.

"He talked on and on about the bylaws and how the corporation could be structured—" Gary was grinning. "Finally, I just said, 'Shit, Todd. I don't care about any of that stuff. I'm in love!'"

I think that was the first time I had ever heard Gary swear, and I laughed. "What did he say to that?"

"What could he say? I was hopeless. He congratulated me and we set another date to talk about incorporating."

We looked at each other and grinned, while the sounds of a busy kitchen wafted out from the back along with the mouth-watering smells of grilling salmon and steaks.

I pulled Gary's hand to my lips and gently kissed it. "It's pretty wonderful, isn't it?"

"We've been together before. . ." He carefully watched my face to gauge my reaction, ". . . in many lifetimes."

"Yes, I can feel it now," I affirmed. I hadn't thought much about my past lives, but with Gary, I knew beyond a shadow of a doubt that we had been together before, more than once.

He told me about seeing the faces of my past lives superimposed on my face at the Fourth of July party when we were introduced. The faces of who I had been when we were together before.

"No wonder you only spoke three words to me," I laughed.

"I never had anything like that happen to me before. I didn't know how to react."

I thought a moment. "I can't explain it, but I get a strong sense we've been together before in Ireland . . . and the south of France. It feels like we shared some wonderful times together in the south of France."

"Yes!" he agreed, "I've always felt a strong connection to southern France. I think that's where we had some of our happiest days together."

We explored the depths of each other's eyes for a time. Then, Gary said, "I've been waiting for you a long time. I'm so glad I found you."

"I knew you were coming into my life but I didn't know how or when." Then, I told him how Martha had described my future soul mate.

He grinned hugely through the whole story.

"Why do you find that so amusing?" I asked. "Don't you think someone could see that my soulmate was on the way?"

"That's not why I'm laughing at all," he said. "I'm laughing because I have a similarly talented friend named Meredith. And she told me *you* were coming into *my* life."

"No!"

"Yes. She said you would be my soul mate. And that you would be warm and soft and you would laugh with me."

I laughed.

"Just like that," he said.

I laughed some more. I couldn't help myself.

"I took her house hunting with me."

"Here?"

"Yes. Right after I decided to move to Washington. We looked at many houses and then we came to the one I own now. I looked out at the lake and I knew I loved it. But I had to be sure you would love it too. That's why I had brought Meredith along."

"What did she say?"

"I asked her, 'Do you think she'll like it?' and she said, 'She'll love it.'"

"And I do," I interrupted.

"And then," he continued, "she said, 'But more importantly, she'll love you.'"

There was a moment's pause. "And I do," I said.

"And I love you," Gary said.

Seen from a perspective outside of time, it wasn't hard to understand how I could be so filled with love—a love of which I hadn't even been aware a few short months ago.

"Now that I've found you again, I'm not letting you go," Gary declared. He took a deep breath and leaned forward. He was so filled with emotion it came out as a whisper, "Will you marry me?"

I was not naive to the challenges of marrying a paraplegic. I see now that Divine Spirit had made sure I would know every detail of what I was agreeing to. One of the last on-site depositions I had taken as a court stenographer had been an intimate, raw account of the daily routines of a paraplegic's life—a young man who had fallen from a dock and become paralyzed as a result. Five attorneys and I spent the day with him. Knowing about the extreme difficulties of that life would have been enough to make anyone understandably walk away.

But my heart wouldn't let me walk away from this extraordinary man. He had been through so much. He'd had an abusive childhood under the sway of an unrepentant alcoholic father. It caused him to shut down emotionally, and that emotional coldness lost him both his wives and estranged him from his children. Sometimes he had been ridiculed by his fellow scientists, because he could see future advances further in advance than they could. Then came the torment of losing the use of his body, of being a paraplegic—and even a quadriplegic—for many years. It had been a hard life and he had weathered the hardships alone. So often, alone.

In that moment I knew my love was strong enough. I knew I would be by his side and he would never have to face life alone again. We had only been together for a few months, but there was the undeniable knowing, a knowing deep in my soul, that we would be together forever. I unequivocally loved this man with my whole heart.

It was crystal clear . . . in my heart. I started to tear up. "I'll never leave your side," I promised. "Yes, I would love to marry you."

We sat and quietly dabbed our eyes. Then we laughed.

"I propose a toast, sweetheart." Gary raised his glass.

I raised my glass, still wiping my eyes.

"Let's drink to our everlasting love." Gary's smile flashed. Our glasses clinked.

"To our everlasting love," I replied, flushed with a warm glow. I couldn't wait to finish our dinner and be alone with him.

18

MIRACLE UPON MIRACLE

As I was preparing this book, I reread the cards and letters sent to Gary by his patients thanking him. With their permission, I am including some of them in these pages. Each testimonial is printed in our patient's own words. Just their names and initials have been changed to protect their privacy. Their words express better than I ever could the work Gary did after he returned from the Outback.

> *I have had severe seizure disorder since the age of fourteen. My EEGs have consistently shown seizure activity every seven seconds. As a result of this, I have been on a high dosage of many different anticonvulsants for twenty-five years [and] my pancreas was failing. After coming out of the hospital for the third time in weeks, my boss called Gary . . . Little did I know then that this visit would change my life forever . . . [After seeing Gary,] I immediately made an appointment with my neurologist and scheduled another EEG. I cannot even begin to tell you the shock and elation both my neurologist and myself felt in finding out that there was no seizure activity at all. For the first time in twenty-five years, I am free. I can swim. I can meet people without giving them a list of emergency numbers. I do not have to take pills. There are no words to describe my thankfulness to both Gary and Robbie.*
>
> *—C.R.*

Now that Gary and I were in love, I was resistant to working with him in his health clinic. We had such a beautiful romance going, I was concerned about being with him round the clock. Could we keep the passion alive? *All day together in the clinic, then all night together too?* As the country song says, "How can I miss you when you won't go away?"

Eventually, I became so inspired by the stories he brought home that I had to join him. I wanted to be a part of it. And I still wanted to learn about how he healed animals.

Since Gary and I had gotten together, my health had improved drastically. I only needed to sleep nine to ten hours a night. I was able to take a brisk walk every day. I felt energized, healthy, and strong. I had stopped needing to see Dr. Giles or any other doctors on a regular basis. So there were no health considerations to hold me back from joining Gary in his work at the clinic.

I became his assistant—much as I had been Dr. Hamilton's assistant—greeting clients, making appointments, and adding a compassionate, calming presence during the treatments. I needn't have worried about the passion. The opposite was true. I adored watching him work on patients. I could see how much he cared for them in how patiently he listened to their story and concerns, in how he responded to them with a warm engaging smile and a soft quiet voice, and in the gentle touch of his hand on the back of their neck or on the injured area. He exuded compassion and it melted my heart every time. I never tired of seeing him work on people.

Doing healing work together quickly became our favorite thing.

It was beyond anything I could have imagined myself doing—going into work every day knowing that I could witness a miraculous healing for someone who had lost all hope. Each beautiful story lifted me higher and higher. My heart opened more and more. It was an amazing time for me.

This was a good period for Gary too. His healing abilities kept expanding. He never stopped delving deeper and deeper into the gifts the Aborigines had opened for him, and there didn't seem to be any limit.

I became confident—enthusiastic—about the work. Maybe a bit too enthusiastic. I dove in with both feet and it set me up to repeat an old psychological pattern.

I'm a very friendly person. I have never found it difficult to chat with people and make small talk. I enjoy putting people at ease by joking and bantering, by drawing out their stories, by encouraging them. Gary on the other hand . . . well, let's just say it wasn't his strong suit.

Gradually, my people skills began to augment Gary's healing practice. My happy, upbeat, positive attitude was raising their emotional outlook and helping them to heal. Gary and I were becoming a team. But my judgmental mind, my early conditioning, wouldn't let me see it that way.

I was raised to be extremely loving toward other people, but very critical toward myself. I was taught that I had to be perfect—to make a mistake was an unforgivable sin. Consequently, I was insecure, self-critical, and judgmental of myself. I was not good enough, smart enough, pretty enough . . . basically always not enough _____ (fill in the blank).

I was also raised with a strict Catholic upbringing—plaid skirts, nuns, daily Mass, no meat on Fridays—the whole nine yards with overtime. Surprise, surprise, a healthy dose of guilt came with my religious upbringing.

Perfectionism and Catholic guilt are not a good combination. Unconsciously, guilt was always running rampant in the background of my mind. And at some level I thought that was a good thing. I thought that the criticism and guilt were helping me do better, be better, that it was my conscience doing its job. In actuality, the hypercriticism and guilt only prevented me from fully offering my gifts.

One day, when I first started working with Gary, I was showing a patient out after a treatment, and I told her encouragingly, "You'll see. Tomorrow morning you'll feel lighter and your head won't hurt."

After she left, Gary brought me into his office and closed the door. "Don't set them up with expectations like that. Now she's expecting that her head won't hurt in the morning."

"Why? You told me you'll be able to help her."

"But she may not be ready to get better right away. You've set her up with the opportunity to fail. She may be discouraged if things aren't as you said they would be."

"I'm so sorry. I hope I didn't screw things up for her." I felt the old guilt clamp onto the back of my neck.

"Don't be hard on yourself, kid. You're doin' fine," he said and squeezed my arm gently. "Just be more careful about setting up expectations."

But my critical mind was on the loose again. Worse, I had opened the guilt gate. And it's Catholic guilt, and that beast is not easy to try to contain. I walked away with that critical self-talk looping in my head. *You're such an idiot. Now you've really messed things up for her and Gary. I feel terrible . . . and you* should *feel terrible.*

I carried that around with me all day, replaying my mistake over and over in my head. Chastising myself. *This is why I'm not good enough to handle this job. I blab the wrong things to people. I'm a hopeless motormouth.*

All day while I was outwardly smiling and positive, I was inwardly cringing from the self-inflicted beatings.

I could have done fifty things right that day. Said encouraging things that uplifted a dozen people. But I focused on the one thing I did wrong rather than those fifty I did right. Where was the encouragement? The acknowledgment of how I had helped that patient and many others that day? Where was the compassion and kindness to myself that I so readily extended to everyone around me? Nope. I had made a mistake and I continued hitting myself over the head with an imaginary wooden spoon.

That night, lying in bed with Gary sleeping peacefully next to me, I tossed and turned. *Maybe I should just stay out of the office. That kind of mistake could interfere with someone's healing. Who do I think I am? I'm not a healer like Gary. What am I even doing there?* I drew in a shaky breath, blinking back tears.

Gary rolled over and instantly knew what I was thinking about. "Making hep C?" he asked.

What he said derailed my train of thought. "What?!" I said.

"Sweetheart, let it go. You're doing a good job."

"But why—?" I realized he was right. I was running a pattern of thinking that had nearly killed me. It was a conscious choice. I could keep clinging to the thinking that had created my disease or I could choose to let it go.

"I love you so much," he said softly and his strong arms came around me.

I let it sink in for a few seconds: *It's a choice.*

I tried out a few different thoughts: *I helped a lot of people today. I'm doing a good job.* They felt foreign . . . dangerous even.

But I kept trying it out. *Gary loves me. I'm where I'm supposed to be. I'm doing a good job. I'm helping a lot of people.* After a few minutes, I sensed that something painful was draining away. A heart-easing warmth was spreading through me. *Let it go. You're doing a good job.*

"I love you so much," Gary mumbled again as his breathing subsided into sleep.

Lying in his arms, I focused on my breathing and letting my body relax against him. I worked the encouraging thoughts a little more.

A strength was spreading through me. I felt like it was possible to heal myself in ways I had never known. I felt . . . almost like a healer.

19

DITTO

When Gary and I married in August of 2002, it was an impromptu affair. We knew we were going to spend the rest of our lives together, and we weren't in a big hurry to get to the public wedding. It was kind of delicious just keeping it between us two.

I still had good friends at the courthouse, and we were planning a dinner party with my judge friend and another couple. It occurred to us we had the perfect dinner guests to act as an officiant and witnesses—presto! Instant wedding.

We didn't tell anyone it was going to be a wedding, not even the judge and the witnesses. I quickly invited my son, Colin, who was now seventeen, and his friend, Bob—who I had informally adopted because we adored him so much—to the "dinner" at our house. We bought the marriage license and a cake and sprang it on all of them.

Consequently, unlike many weddings, everyone was delighted and completely relaxed. Forget surprise parties. I heartily recommend surprise weddings. It was the kind of wedding where the teenagers amused themselves downstairs by pulling wheelies in Gary's old wheelchairs.

It did have its romantic moments, however. As I read to Gary the full page of marriage vows I had written, he became more and more tearful. I was already swallowing hard when I began. "We've both known that when it was time to exchange vows, there would be no getting through it without a lot of tears, because a day doesn't pass when we aren't moved to tears when we express our love for each other—it is so intensely deep and passionate . . . I've never met anyone like you, I cherish you. You make me happier than I've ever been or could ever hope to be . . . I promise you a life of unconditional love and acceptance . . . all I want is to share a lifetime with you, to watch our lives unfold together on this amazing journey . . . I love you eternally."

I had gone on for quite a while. After I finished, Gary was so moved that all he could do was choke out, "Ditto." It was barely audible.

Ditto? Those are your marriage vows? I never let him live that one down, believe me. It became one of our favorite private jokes. When I bought him a wedding ring, I had "Ditto" engraved inside.

Actually, my teasing was enormously unfair because Gary was a hopeless romantic. He was always buying me flowers—especially red roses—and other thoughtful love gifts.

Sometimes I'd come into the living room in the evening to find the lights down low. He'd have lit candles, and a Josh Groban song would be softly playing on the stereo, maybe "You're Still You" or "Surrender." Bette Midler's "Wind Beneath My Wings" was another favorite.

"Want to dance?" he'd say, holding out his hand.

I'd slide onto his lap and nestle my face into his neck. With his arms holding me, we would sway in time to the music—the rising and falling melodies, the beautiful lyrics and the crescendos. Gary loved to dance. I never learned what a wonderful dancer he was until a long, long time later . . .

20

A HONEYMOON

I soon discovered that embracing a life with Gary required accepting a world of extremes. At times life was so full of passion and joy it was almost like a fairy tale. At other times it was like a nightmare from which waking was not an option.

Dealing with a man in a wheelchair, everything slowed down. I was used to a fast-paced life. Now every step, reach, movement, and daily routine took painstaking care. Gary had years to adjust to this slower pace. I was instantaneously hit with it the second we became a couple. At times I felt like my fast-paced life had slammed into the back of a slow-moving train. Apparently, I had taken a lot for granted. Running to the store, stopping off for a latte, going to the pool together for exercise—nothing was simple anymore. Especially travel.

Immediately after our impromptu wedding in 2002, Gary arranged an impromptu honeymoon at the Majestic Hotel in Eleanor, Canada.

Eleanor is a marvelously romantic city, but my experience of it was far from romantic despite Gary's best efforts, because this honeymoon was my first real taste of dealing with the outside world alongside my beloved paraplegic husband.

Up until then, we had nested cozily at his house with all the special bathroom layouts, ramps to the upstairs and down, plenty of space between furniture for navigating a wheelchair, and so forth. On this trip I became aware that every form of transportation, every meal, every stop at a bathroom, every sightseeing excursion would be a challenge. I quickly learned that "Handicapped Accessible" is open to wide interpretation.

Gary had reserved us a suite in the most expensive section of the hotel. In Eleanor, the Majestic was *the* place to stay: beautiful architecture, five-star service, flowers everywhere, and exquisite food. But this turn-of-the-century hotel had not been designed for a wheelchair.

When Gary and I arrived at the concierge's desk, Gary and a concerned-looking concierge had a whispered conversation behind the desk. They excused themselves and left me in the lobby.

I waited for about twenty minutes.

When they returned there was further discussion and frantic phone calls. Service personnel popped in and out while they tried to rectify the mysterious situation. Then Gary and the concierge, with several service personnel trailing behind, left and eventually returned to me in the lobby.

This happened three times!

Almost two hours later, the exasperated crew told me they were ready to take me to our honeymoon suite. When the concierge opened the door to the room and I entered, a huge smile was on Gary's face as he watched my reaction. Red rose petals were strewn from the front door to the bed and covered the bedspread in lush abundance. The air was rich with their intoxicating scent. There were bouquets of flowers everywhere: stargazer lilies, baby's breath, and deep red roses. Champagne was chilling in a bucket with two fluted glasses, and chocolate-covered strawberries rested on a plate on the bed. It was lovely. I hugged and kissed my exquisitely romantic husband.

But why the hushed conferences and the two-hour delay?

I did notice the rose petals looked a little worse for wear . . .

Gary explained it was because this elegant, old hotel had narrow doorways. In the first room, which had been ready for us upon our arrival, Gary couldn't get his wheelchair through the door into the room from the hall. A frantic switch ensued, only to discover that while his chair fit through the front door of the new room, it did not fit through the bathroom door. They had to move my romantic display yet again. After that they had Gary try out every aspect of the room before the move, but those sweet service personnel had set up the room—complete with picking up all the rose petals and restrewing them to the bed—no less than three times!

The concierge asked if there was anything else he could do. Gary asked if he could arrange a horse-drawn carriage ride for us that night. Knowing how dangerous it would be to get Gary in and out of a horse-drawn carriage several feet off the ground, I turned to Gary and said, "No way. It's not worth it."

I was thinking only of his safety, but the concierge mistook my remark and thought I meant that having the experience with Gary wasn't worth it. The disgruntled concierge remarked, "And this from the bride!" Clearly disgusted, he turned and abruptly left the room.

This was only a foretaste of things to come. Beautiful intentions, resulting in painstaking effort, were going to become a regular part of my life.

So many of the difficulties were new to me.

Each and every transfer—from the wheelchair to a taxi, from a bed to the wheelchair, from the wheelchair to a shower stool—each carried the danger of Gary falling. Gary was dead weight from the waist down and it was always tricky to maneuver him from one seat to another. Six-foot-two and 230-pounds is a big man, paralyzed or not. I knew if he fell I wouldn't be able to lift him back into his chair. And what if he injured himself in the fall? We were in a strange city in a foreign country. Where would I get medical help if we needed it?

As the adversities mounted up, it became harder to hide my tears of frustration from Gary. Gary couldn't take a bath or shower because the layout of the bathroom didn't allow access. We couldn't have tea in the famous tea room because the tables were packed too tightly into the room to allow a wheelchair. The visitor center on the waterfront was only reachable by descending a flight of steps. We had to enter the hotel restaurant through the kitchen. We couldn't enter the antique shops because they had little curbs at the base of the doorways to keep the rainwater from running in off the sidewalks.

I quickly realized how totally different my life was going to be. I should have known it would be. I had taken that deposition—of the young man who fell from a dock and ended up paraplegic—before I had ever met Gary. After recording every detail of that unfortunate young man's daily routines and the tremendous obstacles he faced, the five attorneys and I had left his house in shock. Of all the things I had forgotten with my memory loss, I remembered that particular deposition with crystal clarity.

There aren't any accidents. I have no doubt I was assigned to that deposition because I needed to be aware of the choice I was making in committing to a life with Gary.

In all the difficulties we faced together, I never ever questioned that I was meant to be with him. Loving a paraplegic was not something I had bargained for, but after I fell in love with Gary, his wheelchair and every struggle it entailed was irrelevant to me. Part of the package. It was a choice I willingly made—this is the power of love.

21

HEALING OF A SKEPTIC

In 2002, doctors found a tumor the size of a golf ball in my husband's brain [eventually, they found three] . . . Doctors offered no hope, only saying they were surprised Scott had lived as long as he already had. . . . Scott and I went to see Dr. Holz. We were skeptical, but willing to try anything. From the very first visit our skepticism was eliminated by the improvement in Scott's symptoms . . .

—N.B.

One day in 2002, a handsome young couple came to us with a heart-breaking story. They had been planning to marry. The wedding date had been set. The whole family was ready to see them start out their new wonderful life together.

As all this was moving forward, the young man, Scott, decided to see a doctor about the headaches that had been plaguing him. The headaches had started about three years before, but now they had grown to a steady pain and sensation of pressure in his head. The CAT scan and MRI showed three brain tumors. Inoperable. The tumors were in a location of the brain that made surgical removal impossible. There was nothing Western medicine could offer to prolong or improve Scott's life, not even chemotherapy or radiation. The prognosis was bleak: six months, twelve months at most. The wedding was canceled.

But then, after much discussion with each other and their families, Natalie (the pretty blond bride) took a stand. She wanted to marry the man she loved no matter what, even if it meant only six months together. They immediately married.

It was the concerned mother-of-the-bride who found us. She started researching alternative treatments and, somehow, she heard about Dr. Gary Holz. The newlyweds were skeptical. After much persuasion, the bride's mother convinced the couple to at least meet with us once. If nothing else, maybe Dr. Holz could provide a little relief from the constant pain Scott was in.

When I met them that day, they were polite but quiet. I could see that they really didn't believe there was anything they were going to find in our small unassuming clinic to help them. I could also clearly see they would much rather be enjoying one of Scott's last days outside together. They sat, listless and apathetic, as I explained what Gary would be doing. Then, I ushered them into Gary's office.

After the introductions, Gary placed his left hand on the back of Scott's neck. He joked a little: "I always use my left hand. That's because I'm in my right mind."

After about five minutes, Gary removed his hand and shook it. This is what Gary did when pain had transferred into his hand from a patient. Sometimes when working on patients it might hurt all the way to Gary's elbow. If the transfer was intense, he would run water over his hand to remove the residual energy.

I chatted with Scott and Natalie for about ten minutes and then Gary performed the same procedure again, placing his hand on Scott's neck at the top of the spine.

The whole appointment lasted less than forty-five minutes. But after Gary had finished, Scott sat looking astonished. He gently rotated his neck. He reached up and tentatively touched his forehead. "I don't feel any pain at all. My headache is totally gone."

Gary nodded and looked thoughtful, his usual expression.

"You don't understand," Scott tried to impress upon him. "This is the first time in . . . in I don't know how long that I haven't been in pain. I can't believe it." He looked over at Natalie, who took his hand and squeezed it.

Gary just smiled as if to say, *I'm really happy for you.* We were all quiet as the couple tried to absorb what had happened.

After a couple seconds, Gary suggested, "Come back and see me next week."

The newlyweds nodded, maybe a little in shock, but it was great to see hope lighting up their faces as they walked out the door into the sunshine. It was a very different couple that left that day. They were looking at a new world.

When we went to see Dr. Holz, we hoped for alleviation of symptoms, or possibly shrinking of the tumors. We did not expect that in a short time the symptoms would entirely dissipate. After a month of treatment, Scott went in for a new scan. The doctor handed him the x-ray and asked him what he saw. Scott saw nothing and said so. "Neither do I," said the doctor. All three "untreatable" tumors were gone.

—N.B.

22

THE POWER
OF A FOCUSED MIND

After work, my favorite part of the day was cuddling in bed. When we were lying in bed together, the wheelchair was gone. Gary and I were just like any other couple in love. We would spend hours in the evening after work, lying in bed, caressing and talking. I would cuddle up to his left side and fit my head in the crook of his shoulder. My body fit into his perfectly like the pieces of a puzzle.

That day we had seen Scott, the young man with brain tumors, and Gary was telling me what his experience had been while working on him. "The brain fascinates me. I saw the neurons in his brain flashing."

"Tell me more."

"I heard the clicking of the synapses . . . there were thousands."

"What else?" Even though we talked for hours, I always had to draw Gary out. He often playfully teased me because he knew I was so curious about his healing—how he did it and how he perceived it.

"I heard the blood surging through the blood vessels." He stopped talking again.

"This is so cool. You've gotta tell me more than that."

"I could smell the iron in the blood."

"So what was going on while you were working on him?"

"I observed Julie . . . mmm . . . lasering the tumors off."

"You saw the tumors?"

"I can see the inner workings of the body."

"Can you see down to the microscopic level of the individual cells?"

"Yes, the cancer cells looked like green, rice-shaped pellets."

"I wonder if they really look like that?"

"I can see into the cells if I need to, to work with the mitochondria and so forth."

"Wow! That's amazing."

"I can see the energetic flow of the body. I can see the chakras spinning."

"When Scott and Natalie walked in today, it was obvious they thought this was a waste of time. They would much rather have been out in the sunshine. You know, when they had so little time left."

Gary and I had learned that the results we would see in our patients did not reflect our skill or our wishes. Evidently, the universe is more complicated than that. Whether a patient got better or not had more to do with their soul's journey than our abilities. Whether a person heals or not is out of our hands; there are agreements at work that we know nothing about.

Sometimes the perfect patient would walk through the door—willing, positive, open to new ideas—only to be told that Gary couldn't help them. That type of healing wasn't part of the journey their soul had come here for.

And then there were people like the young couple who had come in today—totally skeptical, without any expectation that Gary could help them—and they might experience miraculous healing.

So that night as I talked with Gary about what had happened with Scott, I wanted to know: "Do you think you'll be able to help him?"

"I think a few more treatments and he'll be fine."

"How can you be so sure?"

"Julie told me."

Julie, Gary's spirit guide. It was easy for me to forget about her, but Gary was always working in concert with Julie. She was his own personal connection to the flow of healing energy, the Source of Life.

For every patient we saw, the first question was always, always: *Are we supposed to help this person?* Gary could not heal someone if it was not their soul's journey to be helped.

At our deepest level of being, we are always in tune with the One-Consciousness, at one with our own highest and best good. At some level we know whether it is part of our soul's purpose to heal. Gary could telepathically interact with his patients' unconscious and get that information. And he could ask Julie, who also was in alignment with the One-Consciousness.

When Gary first began healing others, after returning from the Outback in 1994, he would ask Julie a question and get a physical sensation that corresponded to *yes, no,* or *maybe.* Now eight years later, Gary was able to hear Julie speaking in his mind. They could have full conversations. All through Gary's healing career, their relationship continued to expand.

"Tell me some more about how you and Julie work together."

"I'm looking through Julie's eyes. People are transparent to me. Their skin is transparent. I can look into their bodies and see the organs, the body systems. And together we scan for blockages . . . blockages in the energy flow that brings life and vitality and healing into their bodies."

"Are you always seeing into people?"

"I can't remember exactly when it began—sometime after I got back from the Outback the first time." He chuckled ruefully. "I didn't used to be able to turn it off."

"Whoa! You mean even in a crowd? Out on the street?"

"That's why I would look down when I was in a large group of people. It could be overwhelming. But awhile ago, Julie taught me how to turn that ability on and off. It's a big relief."

"Is Julie always there?"

"We usually work together . . . and with others sometimes too." He paused. I waited to see if he wanted to tell me more about the "others." But no.

"My job is to be the focusing lens," he continued. "Julie isn't able to look until I'm totally focused. She needs me in this dimension to focus on the person with no negative thoughts. No thoughts at all actually— to merely focus on them as being already well."

"And you're like the local channel."

"A little more than that. I'm the physical component, the conduit."

"The human member of the team."

He smiled. "I like that."

"You see them being well already."

"Yes, I hold the intention of them whole and healed. Today I watched it happen with Julie providing the healing energy and me providing the intent for it to heal. I don't 'do' anything. It's . . . it's just there. I allow. I focus only on the wholeness. The illness doesn't exist."

Not everyone who walked through the clinic door was destined to heal their illness. But often when a miraculous healing didn't occur, a miraculous comforting did.

When I first heard of Dr. Holz and his work, an Inner Voice quietly said, "Keep an open mind and heart . . . No matter what. Learn and grow with it." This Inner Voice (what I call Divine Wisdom) proved totally essential in the journey ahead. My husband, Ken, tragically suffered a massive stroke at the pinnacle of his beloved career . . . Through this profound journey with Ken [who eventually died of his stroke], I witnessed deep healing in him—emotional and physical—through the work of Dr. Holz. What also helped to bring me comfort, peace, and hope was knowing that Dr. Holz and Robbie traversed this journey with us, side by side, with deep caring, compassion, dedication, and wisdom.

—C.S.

One of the things a lot of our patients particularly enjoyed was what I called the "peaches and cream" treatment. Gary would send them healing energy from Divine Love so they could feel extreme peace, acceptance, love—whatever they needed to help them get through this time without creating unhealthy emotions.

The patients loved it. There's nothing like being enfolded in utter peace.

23

WHY IS THE GREAT HEALER IN A WHEELCHAIR?

That is the question, isn't it? At the end of Gary's memoir, *Secrets of Aboriginal Healing*, the readers and Gary himself were hoping, expecting even, that he would recover fully from his multiple sclerosis. Wouldn't we see him dancing up a storm in the next book?

Years later, he was still in his wheelchair. Why?

Let me preface this discussion with a little story.

Gary and I were meeting Gary's best friend, Robert, and his wife at a country-style restaurant for breakfast. Robert was the one person with whom Gary was able to really talk. Maybe it was because they were both scientists (Robert was a chemical engineer).

When we arrived, I saw that Robert and his wife, Gloria, were already seated at a table and waiting for us. The place was popular and this Saturday morning it was packed and noisy.

"Let me check the table, honey," I told Gary. The Gingham Cat Restaurant was a funky place with mismatched antique tables in all sizes. I needed to check if Gary would be able to get the arms of his chair underneath the table where our friends were sitting. Otherwise, he'd be cutting up his breakfast at arm's length and balancing every bite over a two-foot trek. Try it sometime. I guarantee you'll end up with food in your lap.

Sure enough. The table was low with an underframing that brought the edge barely above knee height. I explained to Robert and Gloria that we would have to find another table a little higher. "I'll check the other room."

I hurried into the back room and noticed several people leaving a table that looked like it would work. It was in the far back of the room. All the other tables were full. I quickly checked the table's height, while the busboy eyed me as if I had an under-table chewing gum fetish.

I grabbed the hostess and asked her to save the table for us. Then I let Robert and Gloria know and headed back to Gary. "There is a good table, but it's in the far corner."

"Thanks, sweetheart," he said and headed his wheelchair toward the other room.

The place was crowded, the tables close together. Gary tried one route, then realized it wasn't going to work, so he backtracked and switched paths. He interrupted first one conversation and then another, asking person after person to scoot in a bit or to stand up so he could maneuver his wheelchair by. I followed along behind, smiling at every kind patron. Invariably, everyone was always courteous about accommodating Gary's needs.

"Excuse me."

"Thank you so much."

"Thank you."

We excused and thanked our way through the room. Coffee sloshed. Shoes scraped. Waitresses waited, holding plates aloft.

Not surprisingly, Robert and Gloria reached the new table far ahead of us. There was considerable moving and rearranging the table and asking nearby patrons to rise, once again, as Gary maneuvered back and forth (rather like parallel parking) until he was facing, and finally able to put his elbows on, the table.

We all sank into our seats with a relieved sigh. Robert looked at

Gary. There are some things only a best friend can say, and what Robert half-jokingly said was this: "My God, you must get tired of being in that chair."

Gary was a contained and quiet man. He never raised his voice. He almost never used profanity. So his reaction was that much more surprising for me. He slammed the table with the flat of his hand and loudly said, "It's the best damn thing that ever happened to me!"

After Gary's experiences with the Aborigines, he moved from being healed to being a healer. In some mystical and unfathomable way—in some way that even Gary wasn't aware of until much later—being in his wheelchair was a part of it.

I could come up with all sorts of pragmatic, logical reasons for Gary never being completely healed: 1) If he got up out of the wheelchair, he might have felt compelled to go back to his old life. He might have felt compelled to continue life as a financially successful scientist and businessman. 2) If, having these healing abilities, he had not been in a wheelchair, he might have been overwhelmed with healing requests. In a way, the wheelchair kept our practice small.

So there's a couple—make-believe—pragmatic reasons for you.

But life is not about pragmatic, logical reasons. They're too simple.

We can't always wrap our mind around the many reasons behind what happens to us in our lives. The conscious mind is limited that way. It's been my experience that there are answers, but they often lie buried at the deepest levels of our being—at the soul level. And they usually have to do with why we came here, why we chose to become human, in the first place. The reasons usually have to do with our soul's purpose.

One thing I do know is that one of the most powerful lessons Gary taught me was through his wheelchair. Because the limitations of his body took away most of life's distractions. In an odd way, it simplified things. He could no longer be a successful business owner and a nationally prominent scientist with a thousand demands on his time. He no longer had a thousand "more important" things to take care of than to sit and quiet his mind. Being paralyzed allowed this brilliant, driven man to slow down enough to talk to and feel . . . God. Gary taught me it's our choice how many distractions need to be taken away before we develop an awareness that Divine Love is always right there, walking every step with us, hearing every word and thought. And he taught me, not by telling me, but by living it every day.

People often mistakenly saw Gary's twenty-plus years in a wheel-chair as an incredible hardship. But Gary was not bitter, angry, or resentful about his paralyzing MS. He saw it as a blessing. The wheel-chair became his bridge to God by slowing his busy life and even busier mind. He now spent most of his day talking to God.

The remote Aborigines Gary visited would spend up to half their time in the Dreamtime, communing with the Big Guy. It was as much a reality for them as any reality is for us.

After his time with the Aborigines, Gary spent many hours in con-templation too. It wasn't unusual for me to find him in the kitchen or at a window with tears running down his face from the sheer joy of it. He spoke to God for hours a day.

"Failure to thrive." That's what it said on Gary's death certificate. What an inadequate description. Gary was more alive on the inside than anyone I have ever known. I never knew him to cry because of the physical mess his body was in—that was the last thing on his mind. He cried at the beauty of the planet and the amazing creations of Divine Love. Oh, he was thriving all right. Tears would freely flow from the joy of watching a bird soar above the lake and then dive for its dinner. Or the beauty of the trees as they danced in the wind. Gary was thriving from the simple awareness of the paradise we live in. He was feeling and seeing God. The love that moved through him so strongly—the love for which he was a conduit—helped him thrive. It was heart-sourced energy and his soul thrived on it.

I once asked him, "Where is God?"

And he responded, "God is *everywhere!*" To Gary that was not merely a platitudinous mental concept. It was his daily experience. An experience he had earned through being forced by his paralysis to slow down.

"God is All." Gary used to say that all the time. With just a hint of longing in his eyes—a longing that seemed to say, *If only I could fully communicate to you the enormity of what that really means.*

God is All. Love is All.

Gary could not have felt more blessed and grateful. His wheelchair—the very thing that brought so much restriction into his life—had fostered his incredible relationship with the Divine.

24

A SOUL'S PURPOSE

My two-year-old daughter, Charlotte, was diagnosed with juvenile rheumatoid arthritis in January 2003. She would start to cry every time her pain medicine would wear off. It was so hard to watch my little baby go from happy to lying in the middle of the floor complaining of her knees hurting. The morning before we went to see Dr. Holz, Charlotte was limping and very cranky. She cried and whined the whole way to his office. You could tell she was in pain. Dr. Holz put his hand on her back for about ten to fifteen minutes. When he was done, my daughter started to tell me by her body language and pointing, that he did something to her. She was smiling before we left the office. The car ride home was absolutely amazing! She was talking, giggling, and singing in the backseat. We got home and she knelt down on the floor at a table and started to color. She hadn't done this in at least three months. As of April, my daughter has no pain. I would probably not have believed it if it had not happened in front of me. My daughter is more active, eating more, and not in pain because of Dr. Holz. Thank you, Robbie and Dr. Holz, for everything.

—S.H.

Of all the people Gary and I saw during our work together, children will always stand out in my memory. They taught me more than any other type of patient. Nothing can open your heart like a child.

Rarely was Gary given permission by his spirit guide, Julie, to work on babies and young children. *Why? Why would this be?* I don't have any easy answers and it was the hardest thing for me to learn to accept.

During the summer of 2003, Gary and I were on one of our trips to the Midwest to see my family. Since Ann's healing, word had spread and we now spent most of our trip doing healing work for family, friends of the family, and friends of friends. Each time we visited, we stayed for longer periods, working a very exhausting schedule, trying to help as many people as we could. From past experience we had learned it was better to arrange for a suite separate from our own room in the hotel so we would have the space and privacy to see patients.

During this particular week, a couple came to us who were friends of my aunt. Their toddler was fatally ill. They were a young couple, both only twenty-four years old, and they had already lost one baby.

Their children had an extremely rare inherited disease—Leigh's disease. To me, it was one of the cruelest diseases I ever encountered. It's a neurometabolic disorder that affects the central nervous system. With this disease a baby can appear to be born normal. They may live a normal first year. But at some point during their toddlerhood, they gradually decline in health and become unable to function. Within a year or two they die.

Initially, the young couple had not known their children had both inherited this disease. It wasn't discernable until their second child was already born. Then they lost their daughter to it and now they found out their son was dying as well. Talk about a parent's worst nightmare.

The young mother came in cradling their two-year-old son in her arms. He no longer wanted to walk or play—he just wanted to be held. Once the disease manifested, it progressed in a predictable way. The doctors had actually been able to tell them what month their little boy would likely die. And unfortunately there was nothing the doctors could do to stop it.

The father turned to us and asked if we could help. Gary took a deep breath before answering, and I knew he was silently asking if he was supposed to help this child and his loving, devoted family. I saw the answer in Gary's eyes before he spoke.

"I'm sorry. There's nothing I can do. I wish there was." His voice came out a little husky.

The answer was no. The souls' choices, and the journey they were on, needed to be honored and respected. *How could this be? Where was the mercy and compassion in that?* I struggled to maintain a composed face. Who was I to fall apart when the parents were being so brave?

The parents took the news better than we did. They had resigned themselves to their child's fate—and their own—long ago. There was about them an almost unearthly peace.

Gary and I were both in tears as we watched them walk down the hall, the baby in the mother's arms, the husband's arm wrapped around his wife's waist. I will never forget that image. Before they were even twenty-five years old, this couple had to watch their two children die—yet they faced it with such courage, maturity, and peace. They taught me a lesson about acceptance that inspires me to this day.

The very next week, another child was brought to us.

I watched as Kevin held up one tiny Gummy Bear for his grandfather to see. Kevin's grandfather was a round, open-faced man named Fred. "What color is this one?" Kevin asked.

Kevin—three years old, blond, voluble—had just returned from a trip down the hall with me to buy Gummy Bears from the vending machine. I had emptied the Gummy Bears into a paper cup so that the boy could reach in and get them without showering them all over the room.

"Red," his grandfather replied. "Red's the color of the fire engines that make the siren sounds."

"Oh. How 'bout this one?"

"Orange."

"Like the orange we eat, orange?"

"Yup."

Kevin held up a green Gummy Bear and waited.

Right on cue, his grandfather said, "That one's green. Like grass."

Kevin's eyes were opened to slits, and you could see the irises rolling in all directions, completely independent of each other, because Kevin had been born blind. I could tell Kevin and his grandfather were repeating a ritual they practiced often. A ritual for seeing the world. Most grandfathers love their grandchildren and are proud of them, but Fred raised the bar.

Fred was a short-order cook. His wife had died some years earlier. Looking a bit weathered in his late fifties, Fred worked the breakfast shift, then hurried home to care for his grandson Kevin so his daughter, Kevin's mother, who was also a single parent, could go to work.

Fred spent his afternoons being Kevin's eyes, and he told us how blessed he was to have such a beautiful grandson who "saw" life differently from the rest of us. For example, grandfather and grandson would sit together at the base of a tree and explore its bark, branches, and leaves, while Fred explained what the tree looked like and how it moved as you looked up through its branches into the sky. Kevin was a bright, inquisitive fellow, and his questions created a special awareness for Fred of the world—a world most of us forget to be amazed and awed by.

Somehow Fred heard about Gary's healing abilities. They arrived at our hotel suite together one day, hand-in-hand, grandfather and grandson. Kevin, with his toy truck and security blanket. And Fred, with guarded hope in his eyes.

Gary immediately did what he always did with each patient—he silently asked if he was supposed to help.

I held my breath, my heart rate steadily rising. After what had happened the week before, I wasn't sure I'd be able to hold it together if we were disappointed again. I carefully watched Gary's face, searching for a clue to the answer he was getting.

The answer was apparent on Gary's face when Gary reached across and shook Kevin's little hand. "Hi, Kevin, I'm Gary. It's nice to meet you and your grandpa." Evidently, he would be able to help somehow.

While Kevin and I made our Gummy Bear run, Fred explained Kevin's condition to Gary. Kevin had been born prematurely before his eyes had fully developed. He barely survived at birth, having had only a twenty-four-week gestation and weighing only twenty ounces. One of the lasting effects had been that Kevin's retinas had not had time to grow to the back of the eye—retinal detachment. They were unable to sense light and relay it on to the brain.

Although Kevin wasn't aware of it, his eyes were always rolling around in their sockets. Since he couldn't see, there was no reason for his eyes to track together. It was initially slightly disturbing but quickly forgotten in the charm of little Kevin.

Kevin gamely crawled into his grandpa's lap for a treatment. Gary's hand was too large to comfortably fit Kevin's neck. So he curled his fingers into a loose fist and placed the knuckles against the boy's skinny neck. Kevin sat peacefully, swinging his knobby knees and thoughtfully fetching and chewing Gummy Bears out of his cup. It was one of the sweetest sights I have ever seen.

After that first session, Gary had a feeling it would require quite a few sessions to heal Kevin's eyes. We were scheduled to fly back in another two weeks, but Gary was determined to help as much as he could. Although his schedule was already packed, he made time to include Kevin every day.

Kevin became more talkative as he got used to us. I especially enjoyed watching Gary's heart melt as he patiently answered Kevin's steady stream of questions. You don't know *questions* until you've been exposed to the curious mind of a highly intelligent, outgoing three-year-old without physical sight.

One particular morning, before Gary rolled his wheelchair over to Kevin, he leaned over to me and whispered, "Pay attention and watch this."

Kevin was patiently waiting on his grandpa's lap. He knew the routine well. Gary placed his hand on Kevin's neck and Kevin turned his face toward Gary and me. As usual, his soft blue eyes rolled in random directions.

Suddenly, both of Kevin's eyes stopped and quickly rolled to the front and looked straight ahead.

Gary took his hand away, leaned back in his wheelchair, and with some excitement watched for what Kevin would do next. Kevin reached into his cup for another Gummy Bear, unaware of the dramatic change in his facial appearance. A big smile spread across Gary's face as he turned to me and said, "Did you see that?"

I was speechless and kept watching Kevin to see what his eyes would do next. Would they revert back to rolling around?

Kevin's eyes started to shift and appeared to intentionally look around the room. He made no sign that he had gained his sight, but his eyes were clearly working in tandem. By outward appearances, Kevin now looked like a normal little boy.

Gary quietly explained to Fred that he had attached the retinas. The next step would be to try to restore vision through this new connection. It was great progress and we were all encouraged, but time was not on our side. Gary and I were scheduled to return to Seattle in a few days. We had to go home. We had patients waiting for us.

Gary continued to work on Kevin. With his retinas now connected, Gary felt Kevin should be gaining some vision, but he sensed that for some reason Kevin was resistant. We couldn't understand his resistance, but then we weren't living in Kevin's world.

One day, Gary asked, "Kevin, what do you think would happen if you could see like everyone else?"

Kevin continued to play with his toy truck in his lap.

We sat in silence for a minute. Then Kevin got down off his grandpa's lap and felt his way over to the couch using his free hand. In a quiet, sincere voice, Kevin said, "Well, I would have to play by myself then."

All eyes in the room, except Kevin's, met as we exchanged knowing glances. Nobody said a word.

Then in a bright voice Kevin asked, "Grampa, can you get the driver that goes in my truck?"

His grandfather thought a second. "Why don't you go get it, little man?"

"But I don't know where it is," Kevin protested.

"I put it in the other room with our coats," his grandfather said. From Kevin's birth, Fred had always gotten Kevin something when he asked for it. It had seemed like the kind thing to do for his little grandson. He was trying something new.

We all silently watched as Kevin stood there challenged for a minute. Then he slowly felt his way along the walls to the doorway of the adjoining bedroom of the hotel suite. After a moment, he walked directly to the queen-size bed and without hesitation grabbed the bright red plastic toy lying on the bed. He had to have seen it! If only blurrily. He groped his way back into the room where we were all gathered and resumed his place on his grandfather's lap, plugging the driver into the driver's seat of the truck.

We only had a few days before our departure. Kevin and his grandfather continued to come, and during that time some of Kevin's other caregivers detected that Kevin had a little bit of vision now.

On our final day in the Midwest, Kevin's grandfather brought us flowers and gratefully thanked Gary for all he had done. We offered to buy the two of them airline tickets to fly out to Seattle for further treatment. But in the end we all decided it was best at this point to let things settle a bit. Fred and Kevin's family would encourage Kevin to want to see, but they knew that in the end the decision was Kevin's.

Over the next year, Fred sent us some cute photos of Kevin. With his eyes both attached and centered, Kevin appeared perfectly normal. Fred's letters always extended gratitude and faith that someday Kevin would choose to see.

In December I called Fred to check how things were going.

Fred said, "I asked once, 'Can you see sometimes?' And Kevin said, 'Yes.' Then I asked him, 'Will you turn your eyes on all the time?'

and he said, 'No.'" Then Fred laughed over the phone, obviously still delighted with his sweet grandson.

I was learning that healing is not always about what *our* desires are. Sometimes, it's about the soul's desires, and the grand design of everything, not the human ego-mind. Maybe Kevin had been born exactly the way he needed to be. Maybe it was no accident. Those surrounding his life seemed to be perfectly in place, like cogs between gears. Even though there were struggles, they had an extraordinary dimension to their lives. Kevin and his grandfather had been given a rare opportunity—to love and contribute to each other in a very special way.

25

THE QUEST TO WALK

I remember standing in my pajamas and robe next to Gary in our kitchen in Keyserville, watching Gary use the sink to pull himself up out of his wheelchair to a standing position. Over and over. He paused to look down at me—all five-foot two-inches of me—from his manly height of over six feet. He never missed an opportunity to rub that in when he had the chance. I looked up at him, enjoying the unusual view, smiled, and sipped my tea.

Gary never let his condition stop him. In his limitless mind, he truly believed he could do anything he really wanted to. He wanted to walk again, so he set out to do just that. Standing again and again at the sink was part of a daily regimen of exercises aimed at returning him to upright mobility.

After we married, Gary was fueled by the desire to walk by my side. He wanted to walk along the beach with me or take me shopping without worrying about knocking things off the shelves. He wanted to travel with me to the places he had loved most—France and Australia.

Gary was a man who had been around the globe several times while in the military, and he had also traveled a lot for his work as a physicist. But that had been travel for work, and he had rarely taken the time to enjoy it. In those days, he had usually traveled alone, and these foreign countries were merely destinations on his career path. He didn't take the time to go out, explore, and enjoy—he was too driven by work.

But his love for me created a desire to show me the world. Gary believed that seeing the world would take on a different meaning and a greater joy if we were traveling together and sharing each experience. That was the dream.

He talked often of Paris—one of his favorite cities. He had spent a lot of time there. His aerospace company, Holz Industries, was involved in sending satellites into space and his work for the French government kept him coming back to Paris. He found Paris very romantic and actually friendly—in a guarded way. He told me one restaurant he frequented would pass him a menu in English under the table, so as not to alert the other American patrons such a thing was available. He took that as an extension of kindness and acceptance.

Lying in bed at night, Gary would describe in detail the streets of Paris and his eyes would light up. He considered it the world's most romantic city, the City of Lights. His greatest desire was to take me to Paris where we could stroll along the Seine River and visit the same little local cafés he had frequented.

These were the passions that renewed Gary's desire to walk again. Being a triple Scorpio, his will was like no one else's I had ever known. Once he set his mind to do something, nothing would stop him.

He hired therapists to work with him on land and in the water. On land, we equipped a special room in our house to hold him hoisted over a treadmill while he partially supported himself on parallel bars. We covered the walls with travel posters of Paris and Australia to provide motivation. His therapist or I would physically pick up his feet and move them while he was on the treadmill. The hope was that as Gary's legs were being put through the motions, his muscles and nerves would regain the cellular memory of walking.

Our biggest hope, however, was that water would help him walk again. Gary loved the water. He had a passion for swimming. When he was younger, he had swum twenty-six-mile marathons. So doing therapy in a pool seemed like a natural choice. Gary went through a rigorous physical therapy several times a week in the local pool. The pool staff and physical therapists were extremely supportive of Gary's quest. Gary was uncomplaining and determined, and it moved everyone to support him in whatever way they could. They seemed excited to be a part of his dream to walk beside the woman he loved.

If Gary got to the point he could balance on his legs with only a little support, lift his foot up, move it forward, put weight on it and then repeat that process with the other foot, he could graduate to using a walker. He would be upright.

We invested in a top-of-the-line walker. It was kept standing in plain sight in the exercise room of our house, ready for him to use when that happy day arrived. When you see people moving slowly along, leaning on their walker, jealousy is probably not the first thing that comes to your mind.

But as we moved through the world, I used to watch people using a walker with envy—there would be such freedom in that shift.

26

FOUR OUT OF FIVE AIN'T BAD

Gary started accepting speaking engagements to teach the Aboriginal healing principles after obtaining his medically related degrees. He came back from Australia on fire about the Aboriginal healing principles, and everything he had learned (both in school and out) only inspired him further. He had been speaking to groups and teaching workshops for years before I met him. He spoke to many different groups: alternative medicine practitioners, mainstream medical groups like nurses and hospice workers, spiritual groups, and organizations that explored the power of the mind like the Institute of Noetic Sciences (IONS).

After we married I joined him, speaking and teaching.

I remember the first time I stepped before an audience. It was late fall in 2002 and we had been married several months. A local IONS group had invited Gary to speak at their monthly meeting. The Noetic members are a highly intelligent group of inquisitive minds. Their organization explores leading-edge science to increase their potential through higher consciousness.

We were surprised to find one hundred of their members packed into their meeting room to hear Gary's presentation. Despite the large room, they had run out of seats. People were lined up in the back of the room and sitting on the tops of heating radiators and wooden bookcases.

This was the first speaking event for which I had agreed to partner with Gary, and I was shocked by the size of the audience. I was even more intimidated because I would be the one doing all the talking. Gary had come down with laryngitis that morning. *Oh boy.*

It was my first time in front of a crowd and I was scared to death. The topic was "The Five Steps of Aboriginal Healing." I stepped to the front and explained the situation, then launched into the presentation. My voice was a bit trembly, and I didn't dare hold up my notes because my hands were shaking so badly the paper vibrated like it was in a high wind. But I managed to describe Gary's experience in the Outback and then explain steps one to four:

1. Willingness: Decide you are willing to change where it concerns your illness. "You may think you want to be healed, but have you really decided on all levels?" I asked them.

2. Awareness: Become aware of the circumstances. "Here's where you get at the subconscious root of the problem."

3. Acceptance: Accept the circumstances. "You may not like it but you need to accept that this health challenge is in your life for a reason."

4. Empowerment: Take the creator role and become empowered. "Use all the tools at your disposal."

Then I wrapped up the presentation.

I was so frightened, I only included four steps out of the five! I totally forgot to give them the fifth step—*Focus.* How's that for ironic? (The step, by the way, is to focus on the reality you want to create, and only on that reality.)

The group was extremely gracious and appreciative despite my faulty presentation. They had plenty of questions, and it was during the interactive time I started having fun. *Hey,* I realized, *this isn't so bad.*

After that first event I often worked speaking engagements with Gary. It didn't take long to discover I was born to speak to an audience. With each presentation I became more relaxed and gained more confidence. After a while I began to feel exhilarated by being on stage. I loved the energetic exchange with a large group of people—especially the kind of people who wanted to know more about Aboriginal healing.

It was easy to book speaking events with Gary because of his extraordinary talents. Gary and I worked out that I would present most of the material while he sat off to my side working on people from his chair. Once we explained the arrangement, and got going, the audiences were more than happy to have Gary working on them rather than talking.

Many people would come up afterward and say they had felt the healing energy.

27

RAY

I was sitting in an examining "room" with light-blue curtains for walls in the Keyserville Hospital Emergency Room, waiting for the doctor to come back. I put my hand on Gary's sweating forehead, "Oh, sweetheart, you're burning up."

Gary's eyes remained closed and his hand was clammy. I squeezed it and got only the slightest pressure in response.

"Oh come on," I pleaded looking at the curtain, willing the doctor to appear.

"Gary?" I asked softly. "Gary, sweetheart?" No reply.

I was certain Gary was battling a urinary tract infection (UTI). He had trained me about what to watch for and all the signs were there: a fever had come on quickly and climbed dangerously high within an hour, the urine in his catheter bag was cloudy and red-tinged, he was clammy with occasional shaking and chills.

Despite sterilized catheters and precautionary hygiene, urinary tract infections were common with paraplegics. Gary rarely talked about his health issues, but in serious tones he had told me that UTIs could become fatal within minutes and that I should get emergency help immediately. I had been down this road a half a dozen times with Gary, but that didn't make it any easier.

The volunteer paramedics and firefighters of Keyserville had always responded promptly to our 911 calls and rushed us to the local hospital emergency room within minutes, but once we got to the hospital, it was another story. Depending on the time and day, the emergency room could be flooded with patients and we could wait for hours for treatment.

"At least it's not a holiday or the weekend," I sighed. I drew back a curtain and nervously peeked out looking to see if there was *anybody* around.

He was no longer responding to my voice. Did that mean we were at a critical juncture? *Should I make a fuss, let somebody know?*

I remembered a story Gary had told me about how once with a UTI in a hospital in Canada he had asked the paramedic wheeling him down the hall on a gurney if he was going to live. The paramedic looked him right in the eye and replied solemnly, "If you make it through the next fifteen minutes, you'll live. It's between you and your Maker now."

I played that scene over in my mind. I went back to Gary. Bending down kissing his damp forehead, I whispered, "Hang in there, babe. They'll be here soon."

Just then a nurse wearing bright-orange clogs burst through the curtain. He gave me a big compassionate smile as he approached Gary on the other side of the bed. Leaning over, he yelled into Gary's ear, "Dr. Holz. Dr. Holz, can you hear me?" No response.

The nurse placed his hand underneath Gary's hand and shouted, "Can you squeeze my hand?" We both stared at Gary's pale hand. It remained limp and lifeless. That's when I started to shake uncontrollably.

The nurse sprang into action. "I'm going to hook him up to some antibiotics and fluids that the doctor ordered. He'll start feeling better soon." Flashing me a reassuring smile, the nurse began ripping open sterile packages of needles and tubes. He had medicine and hydrating fluids flowing into Gary's barely visible veins within minutes. The nurse patted my arm. "He should start coming around now. I'll be right around the corner if you need me. The doctor will be in to check on him later. She's a great doctor. He's in good hands with her."

"Oh, thank you so much." I breathed a sigh of relief and felt the tightness in my back and chest start to loosen a bit.

A few hours later, Gary was sitting up in his hospital bed. "Can we go home now?" he impatiently asked. *What?*

Gary was one of the most patient people I'd ever known . . . except when it came to hospitals. If it was an emergency, he couldn't wait to get into the hospital and couldn't wait to get out. The Gary I knew and loved was back—ready to spring out of there.

"Not yet," I laughed with relief.

"Well, I'm glad you can laugh. And you're not the only one."

"Yeah? What do you mean?"

"Ray's been having a good ol' time, jumping around like a clown, trying to make me laugh." Gary replied, matter-of-fact.

I handed him a plastic spoon and a cup filled with ice chips. "What are you talking about?"

"Whenever we get too serious, Ray shows up dancing around, making goofy faces, trying to get me to loosen up and laugh. He can get pretty comical." Gary grinned while he crunched down on the ice.

"Ray shows up?! Aboriginal Ray?" This was news to me.

"Yes. Whenever things get really tense, he comes around to remind me to lighten up." There was such affection in Gary's voice whenever he spoke of his Aboriginal "brother." It didn't surprise me that Ray was there for Gary at times like these.

"I wish I'd been able to see him when you were unresponsive a few hours ago," I said, maybe just a little jealous.

"Yes, he's a good bloke," Gary acknowledged with a smile. He dropped the spoon in the empty cup and handed it to me. "When are we getting out of here?"

I grabbed the cup from him, kissed the back of his hand, and replied, "I'll go check."

During Gary's trip to the Outback, he and Ray had become

Aboriginal brothers and they talked telepathically almost every day. Gary told me that the Aborigines he stayed with believed that vocal communication through a spoken language was a pretty crude and ineffective way to communicate. They preferred telepathic communication and distance made no difference. Sometimes I would find Gary sitting by himself laughing. When I questioned him about what was so funny, he would say, "Oh, I'm just chatting with Ray. He cracks me up."

Gary and I were a team, but we were only the human components. The rest of the team wasn't visible to the human eye, but those players were just as real.

I've already talked about Julie, Gary's guiding angel and his healing partner, but Gary had other help from the Dreamtime. Gary was so private about his inner life that even I don't know what he experienced every day as he communed with the spiritual planes. As I said before, Gary spent long hours meditating, spending time with . . . I didn't know who, journeying in his mind to . . . I didn't know where.

28

THE ROOT
OF AN ILLNESS

In fall 2004, I was referred to Gary Holz regarding healing two herniated disks in my neck plus residual injuries and scarring from a 2001 neck surgery and staph infection . . . I spoke many times with his wife, Robbie—who is wonderful and an insightful listener . . . In March 2005, approximately four months later, I am healed!

—H.D.

Gary was sitting quietly behind his desk and I was talking casually with Steven.* We started our chat before I brought him into Gary's office for the treatment, and Steven was a lot more relaxed now than when he first came through the clinic door.

I explained what would happen during the treatment. Then I gave Steven some time to talk about his difficulties. As so often happened, the conversation naturally slid to the real root of the problem—the

---

*This is the only healing story that is not based on an actual case. Any story that discusses the root causes of a disease would have been too private to include in this book. However, the process used in this chapter to unearth a subconscious cause for the patient's disease is similar to dozens of cases Gary and I experienced.

subconscious belief system deep in Steven's psyche that had set Steven up for his particular illness. Once these ideas came into Steven's conscious awareness, he was miles closer to a permanent healing.

While I was talking with Steven, I knew Gary was communicating with him on an unconscious level—asking Steven's higher consciousness for permission to help him. Gary might even have already started to clear the energy blockages, both in Steven's body and at the subconscious level of his psyche. The work had already started, and that's why Gary always seemed to be such a quiet man to his patients. He was busy.

Early in his healing practice Gary had sometimes told patients that he was done after spending only fifteen minutes with them—even though he hadn't touched them or spoken to them about their problem! You can imagine how that went over. It was a real challenge for Gary to engage his patients at the conscious level. Conversation was not his forte.

Working alongside someone with the magnitude of abilities and gifts that Gary had, it was easy to diminish my own abilities. At the time I never saw myself as a healer. I didn't realize, until many years later, how important my work was as part of the team.

Awareness is a very important step for healing—one of the key steps the Aborigines taught Gary. Like fish accustomed to swimming in water that has become more and more polluted, our minds create scenarios, identities, and thought patterns that become toxic—and we aren't even aware of the toxicity. Without bringing the sludge to the surface, our minds are cluttered with fear and blockages at every turn.

Sometimes it was possible for a patient to heal too fast. Gary could clear energy and produce a physical healing, but if the person's conscious thoughts, lifestyle, or habits had created the energy patterns that invited this disease, merely clearing those blockages sometimes didn't create a lasting healing. Especially if a person had suffered for many years, they could be deeply entrenched in their illness. It could have become a large part of their identity and infiltrate their thought patterns:

I am the person who gets migraines, so I'll always miss several days of work a month.

I have constant stomach trouble. Everybody in my family is like that.
I've always been sickly. My mother always told me I was the delicate
one.

Those kinds of thoughts define who we are to ourselves and how we relate to the world. Healing means redefining yourself.

Gary once told his friend Robert that he felt 90 to 95 percent of disease is an emotional reaction to our environment. Sometimes that reaction is to a part of our current environment, something that is happening in our life right now. In that case, we can make changes that will alter our reaction or eliminate the disease-causing factor. But sometimes the cause of the disease is a reaction to something that happened long ago, something we can no longer change or eliminate. That was what Gary uncovered in the Australian Outback with Rose. He had to let go of the need to numb himself, a need that had turned from an emotional need to a physical expression—MS! To be numb was a survival mechanism that he had learned at an early age at the hands of an abusive, alcoholic father. Untangling and releasing that childhood belief was something he had to do before the numbing MS could leave his body.

As Gary rolled around the desk and placed his hand on Steven's neck, Steven and I kept talking.

Steven was one of the many men in our country who suffered from fibromyalgia. (Something I knew a little bit about, but not necessarily about *Steven's* brand of fibromyalgia, as you will see.) Steven had been having a very hard time of it, because fibromyalgia is known as a woman's disease and it was hard to get a diagnosis. At the time of this writing, according to one source, 5 million adults are suffering from fibromyalgia in the United States and only 10 percent are men. But that's 500,000 men! Steven was one of them. His physical symptoms were classic. To name a few of his symptoms: he had pain in the specific tender points used for diagnosis, he had trouble sleeping but was tired all the time, and he had put on thirty pounds. It had gotten so bad, he hardly ever left his apartment.

Everyone's story is different. But often, after a patient called Gary, it was not unusual for the subconscious reasons for their disease to begin to surface. Becoming aware of the emotional components of an illness at the conscious level could have a big effect. It loosened up the stuck energy and made it easier for Gary to clear it. It was my job to help that process along through conversation. I was the mouthpiece of our healing team, a job that came easily to me.

As Gary worked, out of the blue Steven began to talk about an incident that happened when he was a child. "You know, I used to be so active. I remember one year my family was car camping by a river. I was seven. I was swimming in the river in a big pool with my dad. We had swum in that pool the summer before," he said, "but this year the water was much higher and suddenly I got grabbed by the current and swept out of the pool and down the river. My dad followed after me and pulled me out. I was fine, but Mom got hysterical. I remember her screaming at my dad. She was shaking so bad her teeth were chattering. We planned on staying in the campground a week, but we packed up and left right away." Steven paused, reflectively. "My family never went camping again."

I just nodded. Steven was on a roll.

"Yeah. Mom was like that. We always had to stay in sight of her when we were at the playground. She was terrified we would be kidnapped. When I was really tiny—I don't know, I was four, maybe five—she used to coach us in how to tell people what our names were in case we got kidnapped. We were supposed to call out to strangers, 'This is not my real mommy. This lady took me from my mommy.'" Steven laughed bitterly. "Maybe if I thought it was safe to go out in the world, I'd be able to get out of bed."

Steven and I made eye contact as he mulled over what he had just said.

Time after time, I found myself engaging patients in conversation to help them bring the core issues to a conscious level. My job became helping people understand what kind of garden they were creating in their body with their mind. I helped them recognize the weeds (the illness-creating thoughts and beliefs) that were choking out the healthier plants (health-creating thoughts and beliefs), so that they could pull them out and allow health to thrive. I helped them learn how to plant beautiful thoughts.

Bringing in greater levels of love from the Divine was the Miracle Gro.

Our nonstop thoughts and our subconscious beliefs are the plants that grow up and produce fruits of emotions: fruits of fear, jealousy, low self-worth, lack . . . or fruits of faith, trust, joy, and happiness. Weeding and cultivating—that's what the patient and I would do in our discussions. I helped them unearth the core issues buried away, the seeds. Shall I keep this belief or pull it out—let go of it?

It's amazing the kind of toxic beliefs and thoughts that can wash away easily in a flow of Divine Love. Once a patient became conscious of the subconscious beliefs and patterns that were contributing to the illness, a permanent healing was much more likely.

Another analogy I liked to use was that Gary was the snowblower clearing away all the blocked energies, and I was teaching people how to stop making it snow.

29

A LONG
AND LOVELY SONG

The Aborigines Gary visited were not only in tune with each other. They were in tune with all of their land, all the natural world where they lived. And they had opened some of that ability in Gary. Living with Gary was full of surprises. I never knew how his connection to the source of life would manifest.

For example, Gary used to sit in his wheelchair at the end of our kitchen counter. It was his spot. He could look out at the expansive view or watch the news sometimes on a little television we had there. He often talked with God and meditated, sitting in that spot. One holiday season, someone gave us a poinsettia, a small normal-size poinsettia like you see everywhere at Christmastime. I put it on the counter next to where Gary usually sat. That thing became huge—three feet across, three feet high! It started out a foot tall, and before I knew it, it was a tree. I just never knew what I was going to see happen in Gary's proximity.

We always had a lot of animals hanging around the house, because they loved the energy Gary emitted. The wild birds would always come to the nearby trees singing during the days or hooting through the nights. And coyotes would come right up to the door. We heard them yipping in the night. They were always leaving scat on the back stoop, so we would know they had been there.

Like the Aborigines, Gary could telepathically communicate with animals as well as people. One time Gary and I were walking—well, I was walking, he was rolling—along a path through some woods and I noticed a bald eagle in a tree behind us. We went a little farther, and the eagle moved to the next tree. It kept stopping in the trees, a little closer, then a little farther back. After a while, it was clear it was following us.

So I turned to Gary and said, "Okay. What's going on?"

"What do you mean?"

"Gary, there's an eagle following us."

"Well . . . we're just chatting." Yeah, I never knew with Gary. If I didn't ask him, he wouldn't say anything.

"What's he saying?"

"Well, he's really very respectful. He's calling me 'sir.'"

In addition to our outside animal visitors, we always had a houseful of everything—dogs, cats, birds. Of course, when I moved in I brought my springer spaniel, Checkers, and my cat, Scooter, but I kept adding to the collection as time went on. With my love of animals, Gary used to say we were going to end up with an ark.

In the kitchen we had our enormous cockatiel cage. We found the first cockatiel—a female we named Buns—on the front porch. We rescued her and then we bought a mate for her. Those cockatiels had it good, let me tell you. The birds had fresh-cut branches placed through the top of the cage and the doors were always open. They had the run of the house and they would sit on the shoulders of whoever would let them—that was often Gary. Or sometimes the accommodating dogs.

When the cockatiels had chicks and it was time for the chicks to go to new homes, Gary would prepare the parents by telling them about it telepathically. The night before the chicks' departure, the male cockatiel, Peeps, would always sing a very long and lovely song—for at least ten minutes. Except for these times, I never heard Peeps sing more than a minute, max. Gary said Peeps was explaining to his young all about their journey, what they would need to know, and how they would be loved. It was a very beautiful song. The mother, Buns, was always terribly sad to see her babies go. Each time, despite Gary's best telepathic efforts, she was inconsolable for several days.

Right after we first got the cockatiels, Gary noticed me spending fifteen minutes to half an hour cleaning the floor of the cockatiels' cage. Without saying a word to me, he put a paper on the floor outside the cage and installed a stick extending from the cage over the paper. Then he asked both birds to go to the end of the stick to relieve themselves. I noticed one day there was very little cleanup anymore. When I asked Gary about it, he admitted he had taught them, telepathically, how to poop onto the paper. That was life with Gary.

We had a hummingbird feeder and there were always a few hummingbirds flittering around it on the deck. Unfortunately, hummingbirds would accidentally come into the house and get stuck all the time. One wall of our kitchen was a greenhouse-style extension, and the hummingbirds would get stuck trying to get out through the glass ceiling. But Gary and I had a surefire method for helping them back outside. I would fetch the mop we had for cleaning our hardwood floors. It had a long, clean white cross section that must have looked like a soft white limb to the hummingbirds. I would hold it up, and Gary would telepathically convey to them through pictures: *Get on the white limb she's putting up for you.* And they would hop onto the mop. Then Gary would communicate, *Now stay there. She's going to carry you outside.* Then he encouraged them to stay calm and ride the mop all the way outside.

It worked every time.

30

YEAH? WELL, READ THIS!

When you are married to someone like Gary—someone with abilities outside of the realm of the possibilities you grew up with—it takes a long time to catch on to all his little tricks. It took me years to discover the full extent of Gary's psychic abilities. If I ever did.

One day I was on my way to meet Gary, and I decided to pop in to Costco for some quick shopping. (Quick? At Costco?) Well, to tell the truth one of my strong points at this time was *not* punctuality. I was always late. Gary was always punctual. Why do these two types of people always end up marrying each other?

My cell phone rang. It was Gary. "Where are you?"

"I'm on my way."

"No, you're not. You're shopping."

"I'm just leaving."

"You haven't even checked out yet."

I was so busted.

But even that occurrence didn't clue me in to the full extent of Gary's gifts. He had to catch me again.

"Hi. Where are you?"

"I'm almost there. I'm on Highway 17, just coming up to the Brock Street store."

"No, you're not. You're at the corner of Forest and Baker. You haven't even gotten on the freeway yet."

I thought about that for a beat. "Are you looking through my eyes?"

Silence.

"Can you see what I am seeing?"

More silence.

"You are looking through my eyes, aren't you?"

All this time he had been spying on me! Oh, Gary was so busted.

The second time it finally sank in. After I got home, we talked and laughed about it. It was good to know he could see through my eyes. I started inviting Gary to look through my eyes while I was walking on the wooded trails around our house. "I'm going for a walk, sweetie, if you'd like to go with me." That is a special closeness, if you can imagine it, knowing he was with me, seeing the same beauty I was seeing even while he remained at home.

Of course, having a telepathic husband added another layer to any marital disagreements, as you might imagine.

Gary and I rarely fought. We were both very mild mannered. But I remember being so mad at him a few times, I could hardly speak. So I didn't bother. Knowing he could read my thoughts, I shouted in my mind, "Yeah? Well read this!" Then I followed it with the appropriate sentiment, knowing he would "hear" me. The effect was usually lost though, because Gary would look shocked and then start to laugh.

31

LYNN ARRIVES

When you live surrounded by thick woods, far away from the nearest house, you can have a bathroom with glass doors on the shower and a large window looking out onto trees (and obliquely, the front porch). I had just applied shampoo to my hair when I looked out the window of our master bathroom and saw my sister Lynn standing on the stone porch staring at our front door.

I had been expecting Lynn for a visit, but not until that night. It was only 8:00 in the morning, and it was a six-hour trip to our house from the town in eastern Washington where Lynn and her husband lived. A long, hard trip. Over snowy mountains. *Had she made that drive in the middle of the night?*

I grabbed the shower sprayer and started rinsing the soap off myself, giving quick glances out the window to keep track of what Lynn was doing.

Lynn was acting so strangely. She put her hand up to the doorbell, but didn't actually touch it. She hesitated a long time and then quickly pulled her hand away, covering her mouth with it. Then, she reached out with her other hand slowly until it was a few inches away from the bell. She held the pose for a few seconds and then snatched *that* hand back and shoved it in her bright blue raincoat pocket. She stood there like a blue statue, one hand in her pocket, one hand holding her mouth, staring at the bell.

Her dog Tex, a skinny German shorthaired pointer, had his nose pressed against the glass window next to the door. His little tail was a wagging metronome.

Maybe the bell's broken, I thought.

I grabbed the knob and turned off the shower. Out of the corner of my eye, I saw Lynn turn and take a few steps away from the door. *Oh heck! Is she leaving? Maybe she thinks it's too early.* But no, she stopped and stared down at the stone pathway. Then she turned and slowly walked back to our front door as if half dazed. Pausing for only a second this time, she abruptly pivoted and headed toward her Honda parked a few feet away in the gravel driveway.

Darn it! She's going to drive away!

I wrapped a towel around myself without drying and headed for the front door. Gary was still sleeping peacefully in our big bed, and I took the long, loping strides of someone trying to hurry and be quiet at the same time through our bedroom, leaving wet tracks across the carpet.

Holding the towel around my still wet body, I opened the front door and yelled out. My dog Checkers was at my heels. Lynn was standing beside her car and Tex was dutifully at her side, looking confused, but ready to jump back in the car and flee if that was the program.

"Lynn, hi!" I said with the usually big, family-greeting grin on my face. She didn't move immediately, so I continued on, "I'm so excited! You made it across the mountains quick. I didn't think you'd even be on the road yet."

She stood by the side of her car and didn't budge. Eventually, she looked up and when our eyes met she exploded into tears.

"What's wrong?!" I asked.

"I can't do this to you guys," she choked out.

"Do what?" Still-soapy water was dripping from my hair. I wiped some out of my eye.

"Pull you and Gary into this mess with me and Sam!"

Sam was Lynn's husband. Now I was getting a clue as to what might be going on here. The last time Lynn had visited us, it was ostensibly to support one of my other sisters, Melinda, while Melinda got some healing treatments from Gary. But as Gary immediately intuited, it was Lynn who really needed the support. During a walk through the woods near our house, Lynn had confided to our sister and me that she knew she needed to leave her emotionally unavailable husband. I'm sure Gary had been silently supporting her in the background—while she made her decision, during the visit and ever since.

Lynn started crying harder. I let Checkers brush past me and he went to nudge her leg. Tex shoved his nose into her palm, giving her the occasional slobbery kiss.

"Don't be silly. Come on in," I said, beckoning her with my free hand. I was still standing at the front door, naked except for the bath towel, but she refused to move.

"I don't want to drag you and Gary into this," she said. "It's my mess." It was that old specter, guilt. *How can I hurt the people I love? How can I burden them with my problems?* Her tears stopped and an expression of pain mixed with courage crossed her face.

I walked barefoot out onto the cold paving stones. "It doesn't matter." I put my arms around her, pinning the towel between us and we exchanged a long hug. Eventually, Lynn pulled back and drew a tissue from her pocket. I had left damp patches here and there on her coat.

"It's gonna be all right. Come inside," I said. Holding the towel with one hand while the other arm wrapped around her shoulder, I steered her to the door as Tex and Checkers frisked excitedly around us.

After I had pulled on my thick navy-colored robe and gotten us both something warm to drink, I motioned for her to sit next to me on my couch in the living room. "Okay. Tell me what happened. I thought you weren't leaving until later today."

Lynn opened her mouth but immediately was choked up again. I extended a tissue box to her and wrapped my arm around her. We huddled together like kids until she was calm enough to speak again.

"When I told Sam I was leaving him, he got mad. Really mad. He grabbed an armful of my clothes and threw them in my car and told me, 'Then get out! Right now!' I was so afraid. I left at two o'clock this morning, and I drove straight here all night."

"You're here now," I tried to reassure her. Lynn is a beautiful woman, a freckled dark-haired Snow White, with a ready laugh and warm brown eyes. It killed me to see her in so much pain. We sat there on the couch and I held her as she continued to sob and vent the emotions of what she had been through in the early hours of the morning.

"I don't care about my clothes or any of our stuff. But Sam wouldn't let me take any of Nate's baby pictures or the gifts Nate made me when he was little," she continued, the tears resuming. Nate was their son, now grown and out of the house.

"Thankfully you've got Tex. I know how much Tex means to you." I looked over at Tex nuzzling Lynn's leg, trying his best to comfort her.

"Yeah, I've got Tex," she said, her voice softening. She reached down and rubbed Tex's neck under his leather collar making his dog tags jingle.

"And you've got us. You can stay with us as long as you like. We'd love to have you." I gave her a reassuring squeeze.

"I feel like such a burden." Lynn grabbed about the twentieth tissue from the quickly depleting box.

"We would be thrilled to have you stay here. You know Gary's gonna love having you around," I said with absolute confidence.

"Are you sure I won't be in the way? I don't want to invade your privacy."

"Are you kidding? This place is huge. We'll have the upstairs and you can have the entire lower level of the house to yourself. It's got a great view, and we rarely even go down there." This was a good idea. I could feel it. I had that deep peace about it that comes from knowing the universe is arranging something for everyone's best outcome. I smiled encouragingly.

Lynn gave a deep, heavy sigh. "Okay," she replied with trepidation, "but you have to let me repay you both." I could hear the guilt in her voice. We'd all been blessed with deep layers of guilt.

"We're cut from the same cloth, my dear sister. I know you'll feel better if you can help out," I said. "And, fortunately, we really need it."

It was April of 2005. Our healing practice had grown by leaps and bounds since 2002. I could barely keep up with maintaining the appointment book, let alone all the accounting and other details of running a small business. "Our business is taking off like crazy and it's more than I can handle. Maybe we can put your superb business management skills to work here," I said.

I saw relief wash across Lynn's face. "I'd love to help with your work."

"Great. 'Cause we could sure use an extra pair of hands." I gave her another big hug. "But we can talk about that later. I'm so glad you and Tex are here." Now *my* voice cracked as I said, "I love you so much."

I wrapped my arms around the blessing that was my sister and held her for a long minute. I had no idea how much of a blessing she was going to be for us over the next two years—another proof of how perfectly Divine Love arranges our lives.

32

REMOTE HEALING

This summer a calico female cat showed up on our deck. She was very thin and lifeless. We took her to our vet where she was diagnosed with feline leukemia. It was suggested that we put her down . . . since they have no cure for this disease. That's when we sent Dr. Holz a picture of her and he began healing her. Three months later we had her tested twice for leukemia and they found no trace of it. She is a happy, healthy cat today and a member of our family.

—M.B.

"Hi, Gary. I need you to be a hero for me tonight."

Gary smiled at me as he held the phone to his ear. "Hi, Rebecca. What do you need?"

The woman on the phone was a professional singer, a gorgeous blonde with mesmerizing blue eyes. She first came to us for help with her dogs and now she was a valued friend. "I'm performing tonight and I have a cold sore swelling up my lip that's huge. I'm on my way there, sitting on the side of the road in my car. I know you can help me."

"Let me see what I can do from here." Gary lowered the phone, holding it loosely in his lap, and closed his eyes. His chest rose and fell with a relaxed breath.

I could hear Rebecca's voice from the phone in his hand. "Oh my gosh, Gary!"

Gary opened his eyes and raised the phone to his ear, "How is it?"

"It's like you popped a balloon. I can feel it deflating. It's practically hissing." I could hear her laughter over the phone from three feet away.

Gary laughed with her. "Whatever it takes."

"That was pretty cool, Gary. Thanks!"

"You're welcome."

"I'm off. See you soon."

"Knock 'em dead tonight," Gary said as he hung up the phone and turned to me smiling.

Initially, Gary treated patients in our clinic by placing his left hand physically on the patient, either on the injured area or on their neck at the base of the skull. He had shown me anatomical charts that illustrated the flow of nerves from the brain, down the spinal column and into the various organs and limbs. You can see a similar chart in almost any doctor's office.

Gary was in awe of the power of our brains to affect healing. So it was only natural that the path from the brain into the body was the path he would usually use. Gary would increase the flow of healing energy to the problem area and accelerate the body's natural healing ability. Actually, the healing energy had an intelligence of its own. It knew where to go and what to do once it got there.

Gary could also connect to his patients on a subconscious level. He could access the subconscious and identify belief systems that contributed to the problem. He could then loosen those old thought patterns and energetically create new patterns.

With rare exceptions, the patients were not aware of the work he was doing with their subconscious mind. Autistic people were one of the exceptions. The few autistic patients we had were able to freely converse with Gary telepathically and seemed to be aware of his work on all levels.

As Gary worked on the health challenges from the unconscious side, I came at the same problems from the conscious side, sometimes following up with e-mails and phone conversations. Often a patient would experience a major shifting of attitude or outlook along with a shift in the physical situation. They would begin to release sabotaging beliefs without even knowing it consciously.

However, Gary had an unbreakable rule: he had to have permission from their subconscious before he entered the confines of a person's mind. He would never work in a person's subconscious without their subconscious's permission and the permission of their higher consciousness. It would be an unthinkable intrusion to change anything at the subconscious level without their agreement. And only their higher consciousness could know the message behind the disease and whether it was time to intervene in the purpose the disease had been serving.

After years of connecting to people and animals telepathically, Gary found he didn't need to touch them to channel healing energy into them. He could help others from a distance and how far the distance might be didn't matter in the least. It's called "remote healing."

At first we would ask for a photograph of the patient. Through concentrated focus on the patient's photograph, he could project the healing energy to them regardless of where he or they were located. He discovered this method was just as effective as if they were sitting in the room with him.

Some patients, for their own assurance or belief system, needed Gary's physical presence. So Gary would have them visit him at the clinic, where he would graciously accommodate their need and physically touch the injured site or the back of their neck.

It wasn't long before we made the natural progression to not even needing a photograph of the patient. With the help of his guiding angel, Julie, Gary was able to go right to the patient with only a first name and a city. Divine Intelligence knew who was asking. That is the nature of Divine Intelligence. It was our own limited thinking we had to get over.

Gary's telepathic abilities seemed to steadily increase. Perhaps they had been increasing since the episode he describes in his first book—when the Aboriginal girl "heard" him thinking how beautiful she was and turned around to give him an appreciative smile.

One time, when we were on a trip to the Midwest to work on family, I was taking a shower in the hotel while Gary rested on the bed. I had my eyes closed, shampooing my hair, and I saw a bright light in a distinct shape behind my eyelids. It was a light creating the shape of a human eye in shades of white with a dark gray outline, and it was pulsating. It was so obviously not something I was making up, nor an effect of having looked at something in the room. I stopped lathering my hair and watched with fascination as this white eye-shape continued to pulsate. Suddenly, I knew. It was Gary working on me from the bed in the other room.

"Were you just working on me while I was in the shower?" I asked as I entered, toweling my hair.

He started laughing in his quiet manner. "Yes."

"You are so busted," I said.

I noticed the pulsing, eye-shaped light often after that. Gary was always working on me in spare moments. Since we had married, I'm sure Gary had been busy making certain the hepatitis C was cleared from my body and channeling healing energy through me whenever he thought I was tired or run down. I had not suffered hepatitis C–related symptoms for many years now. My liver and other organs were healthy.

Gary also worked on Lynn who was living and working with us. One time, I asked Lynn if she knew when Gary was working on her.

"Yes."

"How do you know?"

"When I close my eyes, if he's sending me healing energy, there's an impression I see in a special shape."

"Here—draw it," I said, pulling over a corner of the newspaper.

"It's like an eye," she said, drawing two arcing lines with a circle in the center.

"That's exactly what I see!" I said.

As the years went by, Gary worked continually on all my relatives and myself, clearing whatever physical difficulties we might be having. For example, he continued to work on Ann remotely, keeping her vision clear. It became a family joke: that if Gary died, the entire family would fall like dominos. (That turned out not to be what happened at all, but I won't get ahead of myself.)

Being able to work on patients at his convenience using only their photographs, Gary was able to take on more patients, and we began helping people globally. With the Internet and word of mouth, we started working with patients from locations as diverse as Japan, France, the Philippines, and Australia.

Stacks of patient files in plastic crates soon lined the long forest-green marble island in the kitchen. When a new patient called, I took down the basics: name, location, and ailment. Trotting off to Gary, I would ask the first question that had to be asked each and every time: "Are we supposed to help this person?" Most of the time we were given the clearance to help.

Obviously, my job of helping people become consciously aware of the thoughts, beliefs, and actions that were underlying their illness became much more difficult. With the different time zones and languages, communicating clearly was often accomplished painstakingly on my part with long e-mails or late-night phone calls.

Picture me hanging up the phone after a long talk in the middle of the night, because a patient in France needed to talk before going to work at 10:00 in the morning their time—that's 2:00 in the morning our time! Clearly Gary had a much easier time than I did with his instant connection.

Eventually, we decided to close the Benton clinic and work on patients remotely from our house. We never advertised. Our clinic and house were in a remote small town in the wilds of the Pacific Northwest, but somehow people who needed Gary's help found him. Word of mouth kept our schedule as full as we could manage.

Gary and I found that remote healing could be just as rewarding as when we had seen patients in the office every day.

Nelson is a twenty-nine-year-old Shetland pony who had severe hearing loss and was blind for the past fifteen years. Having veterinarians and horseshoers work on him was a big ordeal because he couldn't see or hear them. I asked Dr. Holz to help him and within two weeks Nelson can now see and hear beautifully! He is literally a new pony. When I feed or pet him, he no longer jumps from surprise that I'm there. He's very calm and very happy. This is quite a miracle. Thank you from the bottom of my heart . . . and Nelson's.

—S.P.

33

CHECKER HELPING

During the winter of 2006 we had a terrific storm. It had first snowed and then rained. But the temperatures had hovered just above freezing, so the snow didn't melt. It soaked up the water like a sponge.

I lay in bed one night listening to the wind howl around the eaves. I was picturing the fifty-foot-tall evergreens around the house laden with heavy snow soaked by the rain that had followed. The wind had come up, and there was a constant plop and ping of debris and pinecones against the roof over my head. Every so often I heard a heavier branch skitter across the shingles. The ground was saturated, and with the wind gusting like this—it was the perfect combination to bring limbs and trees crashing down. Gary was sleeping peacefully beside me.

Oh for heaven's sake, monkey mind, go to sleep.

As I rolled over determined to do just that . . . there was the sound of something enormous cracking and tearing and . . . Boom! With a sound like an explosion accompanied by a huge crash of shattering wood, a tree trunk crashed through the bedroom ceiling.

Thankfully no one was hurt. But I didn't get much sleep that night.

Next day, I contacted Randy, a contractor who was recommended by a friend of ours. Randy came out right away and said he would try to get it repaired as fast as possible, because he knew we had to keep sleeping in the bedroom. We needed the equipment fastened to the ceiling to get Gary in and out of bed. (At least the equipment still worked.)

When I was building my house with Aaron in Benton, each setback left me stressed and angry at the inconvenience and the expense. I felt helpless, I felt victimized by circumstances. But as I set about arranging for our house to be repaired this time, I noticed I was looking at things differently.

There are no accidents.

The Aborigines' lesson had finally sunk in: Everything has a purpose and nothing is random. The Big Guy has it all working together, like a great symphony.

So now, I was actually curious to see why this happened and how it would play out. This was a big deal—a tree crashing into your bedroom, for Pete's sake—but for some reason it needed to come into our lives. And I found out—it did. It was needed in a surprising way later on. However, this was going to be one of those times when I didn't get to know the significance until a long time later.

Meanwhile, I had to learn to sleep with a tree banging on my bedroom wall. The repairs would not be completed for several months and during the first week, the wind was still high and gusty, and there was a branch situated in the perfect way to bang loudly on the wall every time a gust hit. Of course, it was on the wall inaccessible from the deck.

Every time the limb banged the wall, I woke up. Gary, on the other hand, slept like a baby all night long.

"How on Earth can you sleep through that banging?" I asked him—grumpily—over breakfast one morning.

"The problem isn't the banging," he said. "It's what your mind makes of it."

Hmmm.

The problem isn't the banging. It's what my mind makes of it. So what else could I make of it?

My thing is dolphins. I love them. So as I turned out the light that night, I pretended the dolphins were playing a game of water polo right outside my room. The goal was my bedroom wall. Every time there was a thump, they'd scored a point. I imagined them laughing and flipping into the air, dancing on their tails in celebration. With that imagery playing through my mind, I slept peacefully all night long.

The problem isn't the banging; it's what your mind makes of it.

In the following months, Randy and his crew were repairing the house and roof. They were great guys, very friendly and skilled. And what a mess. Every day I let go. I let go of the discomfort of having our bedroom exposed to the elements. I let go of my objections to men traipsing through the house. I let go of my chagrin that their noisy tools were making it challenging to work our now home-based business. It was part of life, a gift. Eventually, I'd know the reason why this was in our lives.

Checkers, who considered himself our guard dog, was not so accepting of the situation. His job was to guard, wasn't it? So he would guard and protect Gary, Lynn, and me from all these men, these big burly men with noisy, heavy, large machinery. The more Checkers couldn't control the scene, the more upset he got. Initially, he barked at the men incessantly. *Get out! Get out! You don't belong here. I will never quit. I will never surrender. So get out, you ruffians! Get out!*

I knew he was just freaked out, so I spent a lot of time patting and reassuring him. Then I got a brilliant idea. I knew Checkers loved to help. Somehow, I managed to communicate to Checkers that the construction project was worthy and necessary and that rather than try to prevent it, he should help.

What a mistake.

I don't think Checkers thought of himself as a dog. He never really understood he was in a body that was limited in its ability to assist with human projects. He always wanted to help. In fact, he was convinced things couldn't, wouldn't, and certainly shouldn't get done without his help. This was a big task—repairing the bedroom—and he'd have to double up on his helping.

The more Checkers tried to help, the bigger the mess he created.

He was in the middle of whatever the men were doing, tripping them when they were carrying things, dancing around in front of them as they walked, participating in the job with his tail wagging and filled with enthusiasm.

Eventually, Gary telepathically assigned him the job of guarding the front door and alerting us when people arrived. Checkers took the job up with enthusiasm. It kept him busy and it got him out of the way.

After that, it became a family joke. Whenever we were trying to help, but actually making more of a mess, my family and I would say, "Oh sorry, guess I was Checker helping."

34

SPIRIT GUIDES

"Denise was sure excited when you told her about her spirit guide today. How did you know so much about her guardian angel?" After a particularly full schedule with patients that day, Gary, my sister Lynn, and I were sitting down to our dinner with sighs of contentment.

After Lynn moved in with us, life became so much easier. Lynn took on the business side of our work and sometimes helped with Gary's needs like taking him for a latte every morning (his only vice). I was able to focus on communicating with our patients and spending more time with Gary.

Gary continued munching on his salad. "I could see him," he said nonchalantly. "I was consulting with him during the treatment."

"You could see him?" I nearly dropped my fork.

"Yes." Gary took another bite of salad. He had a little turn at one corner of his mouth that told me he was in a playful mood.

"Well?" I probed.

"Well, what?" Gary said, as if seeing spirit guides were as ordinary as watching grass grow.

"Can you always see them?" Lynn stepped in.

"Yes," Gary replied, and picked up his water glass. He took a long swig.

Lynn and I joked that we had to play good cop/bad cop to get answers out of Gary. We would come at him from both sides over dinner. I think

Gary deliberately played out the most tantalizing bits to get us mild-mannered women riled up. He found it amusing.

"What do they look like?"

Since meeting Deirdre and Karyn (the woman who channeled Divine Mother and other spiritual beings), I had dived with fascination into books describing our spirit guides and angels and how they were available to help us. For five years now, I had attended every channeling of Divine Mother that Karyn offered. Here I'd been married to Gary for four years and I was just now learning the man could see other people's spirit guides and angels just as Karyn could. Unbelievable!

"Depends," he said, with a feigned indifference to my interest.

Lynn gave me an amused grin and picked up her cue. "Can you see my guides?"

Gary wiped his mouth with his napkin and glanced over at Lynn, looking past her right shoulder. He smiled (a little smugly, I thought). "Yes."

"Well, what does her guide look like?" I asked as I pushed my half-eaten plate of salad away.

We both turned to Lynn. She quietly put down her fork and remained motionless as if Gary could see her guides better if she didn't move a muscle.

"Which one?" Gary asked as he cut into his grilled salmon. Apparently *his* appetite was unaffected by the conversation.

"How many does she need?" I joked and Lynn cracked up.

Gary chuckled. "Like everyone, you have one main guide who never leaves your side. Others come and go, depending on what your needs are."

"So what does my *main* guide look like?" Lynn asked.

"They're etheric spirits. They can look however you need them to look." Gary popped a bite of salmon into his mouth.

"So what does mine look like *to you*?" Lynn patiently rephrased the question.

Gary stopped chewing, looked directly at Lynn, and grinned. "Your main guide is very handsome with curly shoulder-length blond hair . . . and loves you tremendously."

"That sounds good to me," Lynn said, smiling.

"What about mine?" I asked, resuming my meal.

Gary looked up from his plate, glanced past my right shoulder, and squinted. "Yours looks like a big menacing gorilla."

I stopped chewing. Then instantly realized he had zinged me good. "You are such a tease!"

Gary burst out laughing. He was laughing so hard, he was barely able to blurt out, "Yes. I am." Before we knew it, tears were streaming down his face from laughing so hard. Gary was highly entertained by the silliest things. He could laugh until the tears came over a tow truck he had seen with giant toes built onto the cab roof.

"Oh no you don't! You are not getting out of this that easy," I insisted. Many a conversation had ended with Gary laughing so hard he couldn't speak. It was one of his standard methods for getting out of answering our questions.

"Hold it together, buddy." I said, patting his shoulder. But it was contagious. I couldn't help laughing with him despite my desire to get more answers.

"Ohhh," Gary sighed, finally ending his merriment. He wiped the tears from his eyes with his napkin and took a deep breath. Lynn and I sat there looking at him, refusing to eat until we got more out of him.

"I don't know, Lynn, maybe we need to hold this delicious dinner hostage until we get some answers," I said, sliding his dinner plate slowly away from him.

Gary knew when to give in. He could see we two were going to be like dogs with a fresh bone on this one.

He took a deep breath and took my hand. In a serious voice he said, "My dear, Blessed Mother Mary often walks by your side."

Tears sprang to my eyes. "She does?"

Squeezing my hand and holding my eyes, he said, "I especially see her around you when you are teaching or counseling our patients."

I had no idea Mother Mary walked by my side. I felt my strong

Catholic upbringing welling up in my chest and an overwhelming sense of being unworthy swept through me.

"Why didn't you tell me?" I whispered.

"You never asked," Gary said, kindly.

Gary returned to his plate and I sat in silence for a few minutes taking in this revelation.

Finally, Lynn broke the silence. "Does my guide have a message for me?" she asked.

"Our spirit guides usually request the same thing: 'Please let us help you more,'" Gary said. He paused for a few seconds, thinking, then said, almost as if talking to himself, "They love us more than we can ever imagine."

Lynn blinked a few times. "But how? How can I let them help more?"

"Just ask. It's a freewill planet. They can't step in unless we specifically ask." Then Gary's playful mood returned again and he winked at Lynn. "Of course, you may not always like the way they 'help,'" he chuckled.

"If they love me so much, why did they allow me to struggle with so much pain when I was so sick I nearly died? Twice!" I demanded.

"Sometimes the most painful experiences are our best teachers," Gary said, and I realized, *He should know.*

Where would I have been at this time if hepatitis C, fibromyalgia, and chronic fatigue had not sent me down this path? I never would have changed my lifestyle. I'd still be working madly for all the things I didn't really want or need. I never would have discovered my spiritual nature and my spiritual helpers like Mother Mary. I never would have met Gary and have joined him in the work that was my soul's true mission.

Here I was thriving in body, mind, and spirit, doing work I loved. All the time, though I hadn't known it, I was incredibly blessed, loved, and supported on *both* sides of the veil.

I still couldn't get over discovering Jesus's mother walked by my side. I sat quietly at the table and let that settle in. I felt immensely honored. I found myself praying, *Mother Mary, I humbly allow you to work through me to help others. Use my voice, my arms, my smile to send compassion and love as you see fit.*

35

GUIDING MEDITATION

I looked around our living room, which was packed to capacity with reclining bodies. There were people stretched out on the floor, leaning back with their heads on the back of the chairs and couches, propped on cushions against the walls, and sitting on the floor with their heads resting against the seats and arms of the furniture. Everyone was rustling and adjusting their positions, getting ready to relax deeply.

By the time I moved in with Gary, I was completely enamored of meditation. I especially loved meditating in a group. But I couldn't find a meditation group in Keyserville, the small town near where we lived. I could meditate on my own, of course, but I loved the power of the group bringing in healing energy together. So I moved from attending guided meditations to leading them. For more than two years now, since the spring of 2003, I had led biweekly meditations at our house above the lake. Word spread and at times I had fifty people crowded into our big living room. Some people who regularly attended came from over an hour away.

I adjusted the volume on my stereo system. I was playing a recording of gentle ocean sounds very softly. I tiptoed through the reclining bodies, slipped into my chair, settled myself, and started speaking: "Let's begin by bringing deep breaths into the body . . . And releasing them

. . . Focus on your breathing . . . As thoughts drift in, let them gently drift out."

It took only a few minutes for the assembled group to slip in to a quiet receptive state.

"Scan your body and release any tension you find. If you find tension, breathe into those areas." Their bodies became limp and motionless, settling down into the chairs, couches, and pillows.

In a soft voice I encouraged them, "Take another deep breath and let go of your day. Let go of your journey."

The room was very quiet now. A thick, nurturing quiet.

"Now focus on your heart space and connect to your body. Ask your body what it would like you to do more of." I paused. I had gotten used to doing my own meditative work at the same time I was leading a meditation. Today, I felt the longing of my own body for more rest and quiet time by myself.

"Stay focused on your heart space. Ask your body what it wants you to *stop* doing." *No more abuse with sugar,* I sensed my body pleading.

The people in the room remained relaxed with their eyes closed. Occasionally, someone would give a deep, releasing sigh.

"What thought patterns do you need to let go of because they are unhealthy and no longer serve you?" My own answer arose: *My harsh inner critic. All those thoughts about not being good enough need to go.*

"Is there a more loving and compassionate thought you can put in its place?" I asked them. *I am designed perfectly for my soul's journey,* came to mind. *I have all the abilities, tools, and talents I need to accomplish my purpose. I am perfectly designed for the life I have come here to live.*

Their bodies remained perfectly still now, listening to their own inner guidance.

"Continue breathing in and out of your heart space." I paused a few seconds. "Ask your soul what it's been guiding you away from that you've been resisting." I had strongly been resisting slowing down my body and mind. I loved to stay busy, busy, busy, and it was hard to let that go. *Please take more time to quiet your mind. Allow yourself to feel the indwelling Divine Presence in the silence.*

"Ask your soul what it's been guiding you toward," I softly encouraged. I was surprised to see in my mind's eye the word *Teach* with a capital T.

After a few minutes, I continued. "See if you can sense your spirit guides and angels around you. Can you feel their presence? Don't worry if you can't feel anything. Just stay open and relaxed."

I was still integrating the idea that my guides were always with me. I was still learning ways to listen to their guidance. I wanted to help others become aware of their presence. Finding out from Gary that Mother Mary was by my side had been deeply moving and I was still trying to wrap my mind around it. I wanted to let my spiritual team help me more, to sense their direction, to hear their wisdom.

"If you wish to, hand over your challenges to your spiritual team. Your health, your relationships, your work and career. Your team can assist you in all aspects of your life. They want to help you more." I took a deep releasing breath. "Allow their loving wisdom to guide you. Listen."

I knew I had to release my worries about our patients' progress. *Help me to let go of my worries and stay in the present moment,* I prayed to my loving divine team.

"Give your divine team all your burdens. Every time they help you, they grow in love. They are serving the Divine in a physical body by serving you."

I found I had no control over the words flowing out of my mouth. They seemed to come from outside me.

"Know you are never alone. They walk by your side." An immense wave of love swept through me. I pressed my hands against my heart and bowed my head, filled with gratitude.

"With an intention to merge with them, use your breath and pull their energy into your body." I gently continued, "Breathe them into your lungs. Feel their energy join with yours and expand into your body, filling you with wellness." My own body was practically humming now with life energy. I could feel it flowing through me like a waterfall.

"Now extend this combined force out into your aura, the energy fields that surround you and are a part of you."

With my eyes closed, I could see we were all engulfed in a bright white light. You could feel the love and compassion. It came from the group and all around us. The power of our minds and our guides never ceased to amaze me. I loved seeing the validating brilliant white light flowing through us and radiating from us.

"Now have the intention of sending this healing light and peace into the Earth and all who live on her. Imagine this healing light moving from your heart into the world. With each exhalation, imagine sending this beautiful light rippling out, farther and farther, until the entire Earth is bathed in this beautiful shimmering energy and light, sending healing, peace, and love to the whole planet."

After a bit, I resumed and closed the meditation.

"Now bring your attention back slowly to your heart space. Have the intention that everything is in balance and alignment in your body. Feel yourself grounding back to the Earth. Feel the Earth beneath you, embracing you. Take three deep breaths to release the meditation. Wiggle your fingers and toes. Gently open your eyes when you're ready."

Most of the group sat or lay with their eyes closed, peaceful expressions on their faces. I noticed a few people quietly wiping away tears. I was always astonished at how potent a twenty-minute meditation could be. It didn't matter what frame of mind or how frazzled people were when we began. They were always—always—transformed into a peaceful, relaxed state within minutes.

It consistently reaffirmed in my mind what the Aborigines had taught Gary: A focused mind is one of the most powerful things on the planet.

36

STARTING BEFORE THE PROBLEM ARISES

Our dog [Henry] had a cancerous tumor in his throat that was cutting off his breathing. He could not go up or down the stairs and he slept all of the time. He had cataracts and was almost blind. His eyes were draining fluid and his mouth was gunky and foul. We were about to put him down when we began taking him to see Gary. Gary shrunk his tumor by two-thirds and Henry was once again able to go up and down the stairs. He had more energy than he had had in over a year, and his cataracts disappeared and his mouth cleared up. Though we finally lost him to the cancer, Gary gave him six months of quality life.

—W.J.

I looked up and met Gary's eyes as I slowly sank into a chair. The phone had rung late at night and that was never good news. I wondered if he knew what I was hearing without my having to tell him. His eyes were filled with compassion.

On the other end of the line was a woman in tears. She was calling from the hospital. She expressed nothing but gratitude. She wanted to thank us for filling her husband's last days with peace and an easing of the pain. He had died of cancer a few hours before. She wanted to let us know.

Yes, some of our patients died.

Gary had heard my side of the conversation. I didn't need to tell him. Still, I said, "That was Harold's wife." My eyes filled with tears, but they didn't spill. I blinked them back. Normally, I was able to take this sort of thing in stride and feel thankful we had eased someone's passing and brought their loved ones comfort. Gary used to say that I was bazooka-proof, because I never let anything shake me up. I didn't know why I felt so empty this particular night.

"You look tired, kid," he said.

"I'm not tired." There was a pause. "If only they would call us sooner." My voice sounded strangely thin to my ears.

When a person was diagnosed with cancer, they generally didn't come to us right away. We had a large number of patients come to us with stage-3 or stage-4 cancer. We were usually a last resort. Whenever a cancer patient came to us, we would never recommend holding back from Western medicine's treatment, because our work could complement any other healing modality. Nothing we did interfered with other treatments. I wished we could work with patients sooner. Maybe even before the cancer developed.

"We help," Gary said, ". . . as much as we can."

"I know everything works out like it's meant to, but I just wish . . ." I trailed away.

I noticed Gary was holding my hand. I wasn't sure when he had taken it.

The part that our patients played in their own healing cannot be overstressed. Gary could focus healing energy and accelerate a person's own healing process, but it was their body that healed itself. It was the power of their mind and spirit, combined with Divine Love (always present and ready), that brought healing.

Gary had taught a very simple equation in his workshops: Mind + Big Guy = Anything.

What if the Aboriginal principles for healing were taught through-out our culture—in our families, in our schools, in our medical centers? What a difference that would make.

My mind ran over some of the healing principles I had learned working with Gary. That we create our physical self. That our emotions and our body are constantly telling us something. If we feel emotional or physical pain, it's telling us something is out of whack. Pay attention! Take the time to get quiet, still the busy, busy, busy mind and listen. Ask for help from the other side. Release and let healing energy pour into our psyche and body. Make the changes in lifestyle this discomfort is telling you to make. Get the message early. Make the changes early. I thought about how much I would love to get those ideas out into the world.

"We haven't been doing much teaching," Gary commented, responding to my unspoken thoughts.

"If we could bring out your book, teach more workshops, work with people who are only beginning to deal with problems—or better yet work with people before any health problems even come up—we could help a lot more people."

"I was doing more teaching early on," Gary replied.

"But then, there are just so many people calling us now. So many individual patients."

"Yes."

"Maybe we should take fewer patients. Do more teaching. I think there are a lot of people ready to hear this. Not only the Aboriginal five steps to healing but also how to prevent illness, how to listen to your body. All about our celestial teams and how they are just waiting to be asked. I think there are a lot of people looking for this."

"I agree," Gary responded.

"Maybe we need to work at the other end of the spectrum. Start teaching how to stay well. I think it would actually take less time and energy to teach really large numbers of people how to stay healthy—create wellness—than to deal with one patient who has stage-4 cancer."

"Maybe so."

"The healing is always there, available to people. It's just a matter . . ." I trailed away.

"Of learning how to access it," Gary finished for me.

"Right. Do you think—?"

"Absolutely. I think that should be our focus. We should do more speaking and teaching."

I smiled. He smiled. I felt a weight lift off.

I didn't know it then, but it was the beginning of the career that I would passionately pursue after Gary himself passed to the other side.

The physical healing was only a part of the miraculous transformation that has taken place in my life. Since working with Dr. Holz and his wonderful wife, Robbie, I have made my life more enjoyable and fulfilling as a result of Dr. Gary's healing gift. I am continually receiving physical, emotional, and spiritual healings as I learn to surrender to the creative source from which I emanate.

—T.M.

37

THE DARK SIDE OF CAREGIVING

We were sitting at the kitchen table together. Gary's hand moved for the box of tissues. It was just out of his reach, and without even noticing what I was doing, I automatically moved it where he could reach it without rising. Multiply that by a hundred small things a day and you have the dark side of caregiving.

I knew Gary had lived in this house alone, off and on, before we got married. Sometimes when he was really under the weather, he had to have a helper come and stay, but he was often alone—before I came along. I knew he had been through so much alone. I didn't want him to ever have to struggle alone again.

It wasn't until many years later that I came to realize the sinister side of all the assistance I gave Gary. Every time I helped him was one less thing he did for himself. Struggling to raise himself enough to reach the tissue box would have been that much more exercise during the day. Every physical act was some sort of physical therapy. Reaching, stretching, struggling—made him stronger. A little like life, huh?

I loved him. It was difficult for me to sit idly by and watch Gary struggle up out of bed, struggle over to where he kept his clothes, struggle into them while sitting in the chair. So, I helped.

I'm a caregiver by nature. It's in my blood.

It was difficult for me to watch Gary struggle from his chair to the stool in the shower, realize that he had forgotten the new shampoo, struggle back into his chair, roll out to the kitchen where he'd left the shampoo, roll back to the shower and struggle back onto the stool. So, I helped. It would have been ridiculous not to.

It was difficult for *Gary* to watch me straining to take his weight while he transferred into bed at night or out of it in the morning. Difficult for him to see me, lifting and staggering, trying to make each transfer smooth, terrified he would fall. And there were so many transfers during a day.

So, *he* helped *me*—by agreeing to buy the special equipment that would take the strain off my petite body. We put a transfer system in the bedroom that had tracks on the ceiling. I could fasten a harness around him and use the machine's pulleys to lift him and rotate him from the bed to his chair, or to lift him while he got dressed.

I didn't know the effect making things easier would have. Every mechanical aid, every time I took some of Gary's weight or fetched him something, cost Gary some strength building, cost Gary some muscle.

Safety versus strength building, it was a trade-off. Even with my help, Gary fell so often we knew the EMTs on a first-name basis and were able to joke around with them each time they had to be called. Any one of those falls might have resulted in a serious injury—a broken bone, a concussion. Daily life was a challenge every way we turned. Any relief from the strain was much appreciated . . . by us both.

I doubt in the long run we would have chosen to do things differently.

The last visit we made to the public pool the manager was in an agony of discomfort. I could see he *really* wanted to be anywhere but where he was, saying anything but what he had to say. He had hurried out from his office to intercept Gary and me before we got in the pool—the one pool in our small town.

There we stood (and sat) in our swimsuits, totally perplexed by what the pool manager was saying.

"It doesn't look safe." He wiped a hand over his balding head. "When you just dump him out of the chair . . ." He seemed to realize Gary was sitting right there and turned to face him. "I mean . . . when you just . . . dive from the chair into the water, it's dangerous."

"But Sarah is right there the minute he hits the water," I cut in. (Sarah was our strapping six-foot-tall physical therapist.) "She could pull him up to the surface if Gary got into trouble."

"It's still not safe."

"You've seen Gary swim. He's a strong swimmer once he gets in. Transferring him on to the lift chair to get into the water . . . that, that's actually the dangerous part." Gary's arm strength had deteriorated to the point that getting himself on the lift chair to get into the pool wasn't an option anymore, so we had started tipping him into the pool from the side. This discussion wasn't going the direction I wanted it to. "Gary used to swim twenty-six-mile marathons," I finished lamely.

"The way you're getting him into the pool, he could hit his head or catch an arm on the side. If we let you . . . do something that isn't safe, and something happens, the city is liable. It has to be our call. You understand?"

Yes, we understood. Even though we didn't want to face it, he was right. The staff at the pool had gone out of their way to help us for years. They had done everything within reason—and even a little bit beyond reasonable. We were very grateful.

And it still was a terrible disappointment.

Gary touched my arm. It was obvious the pool manager wasn't going to be able to change the situation. He was nearly as upset about it as we were. Was it really that surprising they couldn't allow us to dump Gary from his wheelchair directly into the pool? The poor manager was right. Gary could get injured. We had been willing to take that chance, because it was the only option left. The only way that Gary could keep exercising in the water.

We could always hire three strong therapists to carry Gary in, but we all knew that wasn't going to happen. A nightmare of logistics, it was outside what could realistically be arranged.

"We understand," Gary said quietly. "Thanks."

With a last sympathetic look, the pool manager hurried off.

"You get changed," I said. "I'll send Sarah home and go get the van."

"No," Gary insisted. "You should get a swim in. I don't mind waiting."

"I don't need to. It's okay."

"Don't be silly. At least you should get some exercise." I could see it was going to make him feel worse if I didn't swim.

"Okay," I said. "Just twenty minutes."

So Gary watched as I swam laps at the far side of the pool. I was thankful the pool water hid my tears. I knew, as Gary knew, sitting in his dry swimming trunks in his wheelchair on the sidelines of the pool, this was the beginning of the end.

38

A LESSON IN GRATITUDE

That last trip to the pool was in the spring of 2006. I didn't know it, but a few months earlier in January of 2006, Gary's spirit guide, Julie, told him that he needed to put his worldly affairs in order—he was being called home. He would have about a year more in his human body. He was needed for what he would be better able to do on the other side of the veil.

His soul's journey in this body was complete.

It took Gary a few months to come to terms with it. I'm sure there was a lot of time spent communicating with his spirit team trying to negotiate. Finally, he became reluctantly convinced that there was no negotiation to be had. This was what Gary's soul had planned—his work here was done.

Shortly after that fateful trip to the pool, Gary tearfully confessed it to me: He would be dying early next year.

I was devastated.

It took me weeks to get from numb, to sad, to—finally—angry. I was still struggling with my anger when the universe gifted me with a lesson that would last the rest of my life. The tools the universe needed to accomplish this lesson were a set of car keys, and a large open grassy field.

My sister was still living with us and she hadn't had the chance to see the orca whales of which there are several pods in Puget Sound. I had tickets to an orca whale–watching expedition—maybe the last one my animal communicator friend would be guiding since she was leaving the area—and I gave them to Lynn. Only one of us could go.

After waving farewell, I decided to take Tex and Checkers for a walk in the large grassy field we often went to along the waterfront near our home.

It was Sunday, a beautiful clear spring day. *Perfect for a whale-watching trip,* I thought (maybe with just a little bit of self-pity). Across the blue water, the snow-topped mountains stood out vividly against the even more blue sky. I was glad to be there in the early morning as the forecast for later predicted an unseasonably hot day.

As was their custom, both dogs took off running immediately to chase after all the smells that wafted about on the ground. As I had dozens of times before, I locked the car, placed the car keys in my worn brown coat pocket and eventually caught up with them in the overgrown field.

Quickly, my mind returned to thoughts of losing Gary. *How could he leave me? It wasn't fair and it was so unbearably sad.* We hadn't told anyone yet. I was too upset to talk about it to anyone else, even my sister. What would I say? How could I explain it?

As was usual of late, my sadness flipped to anger. *Why now? Why now when Gary had finally found happiness?* Gary and I were so much in love. He was finally enjoying relationships with his son and daughter and the joys of being a grandfather. He had found a warm embrace in my family. We had wonderful friends and he felt loved and supported on all sides. After so much suffering, he was finally truly happy. *We* were happy. *Doesn't that count for something, God?* My cheeks burned and hot angry tears came yet again.

These thoughts circled around my head as the dogs and I circled around the field. So many questions. And guess what? Divine Love had an answer for me. "Ask and you will receive." But not always in the form you anticipated . . .

The dogs and I walked the perimeter of the field in the usual half hour. When we arrived back at the car and I went to unlock it, I discovered I didn't have my keys.

I checked and rechecked every pocket in my weathered brown coat and my pants. No keys! *This can't be, because this would be very bad. Surely I'll find my keys. Maybe they're lying on the ground or they're in the ignition.* I could see the keys weren't in the ignition. I could also see my purse—lying clearly visible on the front floor of the car with my cell phone tucked inside. *Arrgh!*

I started to check the grass along the field. I scoured that field. I walked our route several times, kicking aside the grass, getting on my knees at times. No keys.

It had started getting uncomfortably warm and the dogs were panting. My heart began beating fast and I realized I was starting to panic. It's funny how dependent we get on keys, purse, credit cards, cell phones. The Aborigines manage to live without any of those things. But I wasn't thinking about that right now. I was in the middle of nowhere with no one in sight and I had two large thirsty muddy dogs with me and I needed to find a way to get us all home.

Some distance away I could see an industrial area with large warehouses and machine shops. It was Sunday and the place looked totally deserted, but it was worth a try. With both dogs in tow, I started walking toward it.

But when we reached the industrial complex, building after building was locked up tight and deserted on this beautiful Sunday morning. It was like a ghost town.

Finally, I came upon a man and his son cleaning the inside of one of the buildings. I could see they had arrived in a large van, which could easily have taken the dogs and me home, but this was not what the universe had planned. His son had severe allergies, so there was no way he could carry the dogs in his van.

He offered me his cell phone to call a taxi, but I knew no taxi service would take me and these two large muddy dogs, even if we could find a taxi available on a Sunday in our small town—I'd never seen one.

I thanked him for the thought and asked if I could use his cell phone to call my husband.

It took forever for Gary to get to the phone. (If he was in certain locations in the house, answering the phone was not an easy task.) I explained my situation. He couldn't come get us, because we had let my son borrow the wheelchair accessible van to help friends move some large items over the weekend. Lynn would normally have been available, but she was on a whale-watching trip—the fun trip I was supposed to be on—and wouldn't be back until late evening.

My strongest hope was that my friends who lived down the road could come get us. It took about ten minutes for Gary to provide their phone number. I called them. No answer. I called Gary back and got the numbers of other friends, but again—no answers.

That's when my radar went up. Clearly the universe was sending me a strong message. There were so many odd circumstances falling into place in order for me to be stuck like this. I knew that when the universe was trying to tell me something, it was in my best interest to listen. It was always best to pay attention when I was being tapped on the shoulder—as opposed to being slammed into a wall to get my attention. This was something I knew well from past experience.

But I had no idea what all this meant. When I was blindsided like this, I knew there was something I was meant to learn, and there wouldn't be any avoiding it. *So sit up and pay attention.* But I didn't have a clue what the universe was trying to tell me with this one.

So that morning, I was standing there with two big, hot, filthy dogs on leashes and no apparent way to get home because every possible vehicle and friend had been exhausted, and I'm listening. *What?! What are you trying to tell me?!* But I couldn't for the life of me figure out what the message was.

And I was mad again. *Was this fair? Didn't I give up what promised to be a fantastic whale-watching trip? Wasn't I the one dealing with the impending loss of my husband? How comforting was this?!*

This just sucked.

I thanked the man who had graciously loaned me his cell phone and I continued to walk down the street through the empty industrial park.

A few blocks later I saw people—finally!

I hurried over, delighted at signs of life and possible rescue. It was a Hispanic family cleaning the grounds, picking up debris and weeding outside a commercial building. The middle-aged woman with a flashing smile was probably the mother. Her husband had kindly eyes and a firm handshake. Neither of them spoke much English, but the two girls and the prepubescent boy who were their children spoke some.

After I relayed my situation, with broad smiles and broken English they conveyed to me that they would be more than happy to provide a ride for me and my dogs as soon as their other son returned with their car. The children petted the dogs and everyone made friends. I was so relieved—I finally had a way home with the dogs.

I tied the dogs up to a post and started pulling weeds and picking up garbage with them in the sun. The dogs were happy to flop down in the little bit of shade offered by a nearby building and watch me with their tongues hanging out.

Everybody went back to work. I was impressed with how hard the kids went at it without any complaining. In fact, the entire time they worked, the whole family was chatting and joking in Spanish (of which I spoke not a word). They laughed together every other minute, and there was a lot of patting and squeezing of shoulders whenever one passed another. They never stopped working, but they seemed content merely to be together as a family on this bright spring Sunday, picking up garbage.

Every time someone caught my eye they'd smile, a big genuine warm smile. The boy tossed a little conversation in English my way every so often. I learned that today was their one day off from their regular jobs. This was their *second* job. They all worked seven days a week.

By this time the sun was blasting the sky. I looked around for their supplies. As near as I could tell, they had no water. No food. The lot was thick with weeds among the landscaping, but I noticed they had no tools. None of them even had gloves to protect their fingers as they pulled up blackberry brambles and thistles.

The older girl started quietly singing a lilting Spanish song in a sweet high voice. The others joined in after a few lines, the papa's voice gruff and low. It would hardly have qualified as recording quality, but after they finished (somewhat off-key) everyone laughed delightedly. I smiled around encouragingly. The youngest boy shrugged good-naturedly.

I picked up a bright blue cap like those on an expensive juice bottle. The boy noticed and reached for it. "Felicia will want that." He tossed it to his youngest sister, "Felicia! Mira, azul."

"Aaii!" she said and stuck it in her pocket.

I looked at him quizzically and he grinned. "She has a rainbow. She needs the blue ones." He moved his hands in a wide arc. "Over her bed. All the colors." Of course. They wouldn't have a lot of money to spend on home décor. Kids loved things that were plastic and brightly colored. I could picture the layered arc of plastic caps taped or pasted to her wall, a rainbow arching over the head of her bed. Lemons and lemonade, garbage and rainbows.

Their teenage son didn't arrive with their car for about an hour, so I had plenty of time to think about what I was being shown.

Here was a family who had to work seven days a week. They had so little in the way of material wealth. They had no tools and decorated with trash. But they weren't sad. They weren't complaining. They were enjoying the love they all shared in every way they could—smiling, enjoying the sunny day, singing, and hugging. And generously offering to drive me (a total stranger) and my dogs home, when they had practically nothing.

I had a beautiful home and all the food and water I needed. I didn't have to work 24/7. I had friends and family and a generous, devoted sister. *I have a handsome, unbelievably gifted husband who loves me and I love him.* But was I enjoying all that?

No. I was stressed, angry, and depressed nearly all the time lately. Before this all happened, I was spending this beautiful day thinking:

I lost my keys. This sucks. This is so unfair.

I really wanted to go on the whale-watching trip.

It's hot and I'm thirsty.

My husband is dying in a year.

Wah, wah, wah.

Then I was shown this amazing family and how *they* are spending the day.

My thoughts were interrupted by the arrival of their son with the car, a station wagon that had seen many mediocre days since seeing better days.

Their son hopped out of the driver's seat and there was a quick, good-natured interchange in Spanish. He said something teasingly to his mother and she threw the crook of her elbow around his neck and rubbed his hair against the part. He ducked out of her grasp and smoothed his hair back into place. *Don't mess with the hair, Ma.*

Then the mother slid in behind the wheel and tossed her head, beckoning for me to get in with the dogs.

When we arrived at my house, I frantically motioned for her to wait a minute. I ran inside and grabbed money, water, and some snack bars. When I extended the money toward her through the driver's window, she shook her head, waving her hands emphatically. She refused everything but the water. Flashing a warm smile, she drove off. I never saw any of them again.

The lesson the universe had been trying to teach me became very clear as soon as she pulled out of the driveway. These kind people who had so little to give, gave more to me than they will ever know. They had shown me by their actions, their attitudes, and by the love they shared to be thankful for what I had.

To live in the present moment.

I didn't know how much longer Gary would live. I needed to make the most of every precious second.

We didn't have as much time to share with each other as I wanted. But our love for each other and our families was the most precious commodity Gary and I possessed and we had it in abundance. Both of us needed to stop focusing on how unhappy we were that Gary was leaving and instead focus on what we did have.

Gratitude, I have since learned, moves the energy of the universe very fast. You can turn any situation around very quickly by shifting your focus to gratitude. By remembering what you have to be grateful for in this moment, you effectively change your entire experience of life—even in the most painful of circumstances. Gratitude is extremely powerful, and it works every time.

That was the day Gary and I came to accept his impending passing. We talked it over and took a vow: to move beyond the anger and the sadness, to enjoy our time together, to stay in the present moment.

As it turned out, I had thousands of those precious moments before Gary died. If by some miracle you are reading this—happy Hispanic family—thank you.

39

WAITING

Gary and I always loved talking in bed at the end of the day, but it became a huge challenge for me to hold it together as 2007 arrived. Gary had been getting steadily weaker in body (though not in spirit), and we both knew it would only be a short time before he passed.

Gary kept working on patients during the first month of the year, and I continued to keep the business going. During the day, I was careful not to let him see me cry. I would leave the room and pretend to be going to the bathroom, or I'd hold it in until I could say I was going out for a walk. But when Gary was lying in my arms at night, I could feel him gradually slipping away from me as his body deteriorated and weakened. I hoped he didn't feel my occasional tear running down his bare arm.

I didn't want him to see my unhappiness. I didn't want to add to his burdens and the pain he was feeling from having to leave those he loved behind. In my typical style, I didn't want him to worry about *me*, so I tried to hide my feelings.

One night, we were lying naked in bed together with my head tucked in the hollow of his shoulder, and I couldn't hold back any longer. "I'm going to miss you so much," I said. "I can't imagine life without you." Tears started rolling down my face onto his bare chest.

After a long pause, he said, "I'm going to miss you too."

There was a longer pause. The only sound was me quietly weeping and sniffling.

Kissing the top of my head, Gary gently responded, "You're going to be okay, sweetheart. You'll be fine."

"I'm really scared," I said.

Gary squeezed me a little tighter. "Remember what your guides always say?"

"I know. They're always telling me, 'Let us help you more.'"

"Mother Mary walks with you too. Lean on Mother Mary and your guides."

I felt a little bit of peace, a little lessening of the heartbreak. But part of me was still holding on to the fear of losing my soul mate and lover soon.

It wasn't long before I fell into my old patterns again, looking to food for comfort, eating lots of sugar, salt, and fat. Working all the time, taking care of every detail of Gary's care and keeping the business going, never taking time out, because that would allow the grief to surface. Putting on an outwardly happy, bubbly composure all day long. *I'm the strong one. I'm bazooka-proof.* Never taking the time to feel my feelings and realize they were based on love. Shouldering it all myself without handing it over to my spiritual team, to Divine Love.

What I didn't understand at the time was Gary was still here for my sake. He was making sure every tiny bit of hepatitis C was gone from my body forever. He wanted to be sure the fibromyalgia and chronic fatigue were never coming back. He could do that energetically, but not if I kept re-creating it with my old patterns of behavior and thinking.

Remember him asking me over the last seven years, "Making hep C, are you?" Now Gary was waiting—he was holding back death, waiting—for me to make the final changes. All those things that Gary had been quietly reminding me of while he had been with me, all the things he used to remind me to do every day—I had to learn to do them for myself now.

These are the things Gary used to say to me all the time:

"Slow down, woman!" I needed to get more rest. I needed to slow myself down, emotionally and physically.

"Sit and talk to me." Now instead of sitting and talking with Gary, I needed to learn to talk with Divine Love. To sit and connect with the Source of Life, as deeply and as often as I could.

"Let it go!" I needed to let go, to accept the situation no matter how painful it was. To stop putting all my energy into denial. By asking for Spirit's help and turning it over, I was actually allowing a higher level of empowerment to come into play. My own empowerment.

"Less is more." I needed to simplify my life. Not take care of every detail, but eliminate the details. Simplify.

"Love ya, kid." I needed to stop putting the needs of others ahead of mine. I needed to love and care for myself. And, instead of taking care of everybody else's needs and denying them the chance to take care of mine, I needed to allow others to help *me* too.

In March, I made a commitment to a greater level of care for myself. I slowed everything down. I changed my diet and spent more time meditating or walking in nature. Throughout my day, I focused on connecting to Divine Love, feeling the Presence. I practiced self-love and self-care—I put myself at the top of the list.

Two weeks later, Gary could see my commitment and knew my relationship with Divine Love was strong. He knew he could now leave. Within a week's time his health rapidly declined.

One day, lying beside him in bed, I asked him, "Sweetheart, were you waiting for me to start taking better care of myself?"

His smile was weak but genuine. "Yes."

"It's funny, but by taking better care of myself, I feel closer to God, to Divine Love."

"You are." His voice was soft and the words came slowly. "Your connection is strong. I can see it."

"You never said anything. You never pushed me."

"No. I have faith in you. I'm so proud of you."

He had been silently waiting for me to make the changes in my life. He had never once hinted that was what he was doing. I had to discover on my own that I needed to change. It was just another example of the extreme love Gary quietly bestowed on me.

Later the same day, I noticed the quote on my daily calendar: "No one can persuade another to change. Each of us guards a gate of change that can only be opened from the inside."

40

THE GATHERING
AT THE CROSSING

One morning Gary awoke too weak to get out of bed. I brought his breakfast in to him there.

For the first time, I sat down to eat breakfast in our usual spot alone. I was looking out the window and I noticed a little humming-bird perched on the top of a white flowering tree just outside. I got the otherworldly sense it was Gary. That since he couldn't get out of bed that morning this was him joining me for breakfast.

From that time on, I usually saw this same hummingbird on the top branch of its favorite tree outside my kitchen window when I sat down to eat. Always I felt like it was Gary joining me for my meals. Gary's poor body lay weakened and dying in our bed down the hall, but he and this little guy had worked out a way to keep me company.

Hummingbirds. What happened during the week of Gary's dying, and after, would forever change my relationship to these tiny warriors.

Don't let anyone mislead you. Dying at home is not for wimps. As Gary's body shut down, one of the first organs to go was his skin. He never complained. But I knew he must be suffering. He developed terrible lesions from lying helpless in bed, the skin of his back and legs shredded like tissue and bled as I tried to clean it. My heart ached for him.

This kind of indignity and pain made it easier for me to let him go. Those of you who have been through it will understand. I said I was ready for Gary to pass—I repeated it in my conscious thoughts—but deep down I was still holding on, wishing he would live just a little longer. Watching Gary suffer through those last days peeled back the layers of my resistance, one by one.

Pain medication or consciousness? It's always a trade-off. Our valiant hospice workers—I was so grateful for their patience and sensitivity.

As we waited for the hospice nurse to bring the drug that would take him out of the pain, but into unconsciousness, Gary was still helping others. He was trying to help as many as he could before he passed. He asked for my sister Lynn many times. Holding her hand, he sent healing energy into her. He told me to call my brother Steve for him. During this time—just before his death, but while he was still lucid—he sent the strongest energy I had ever seen. He smiled so beautifully to the hospice nurse when she finally came.

I lay in bed with Gary and kissed his face while she inserted a PICC line (a catheter inserted into a vein to deliver intravenous pain medication quickly). I told him I released him to go to God. He said, "Thank you."

After the hospice nurse left, Gary wanted me to go out of the room and close the door. I knew he just wanted me to have time to relax and let him go. He was at peace. I could see it on his face. It was terribly hard to tear myself away from his side in what might have been his last hours. I wanted him to open his eyes again and say, "I love you." I wanted his last words to me to be "I love you" instead of "Thank you."

He might never fully regain consciousness again. But it didn't matter. I knew Gary loved me. Everything he did or asked was out of love for me. I saw that so clearly.

My heart was breaking, yes, breaking open. During the last week of Gary's life, the messages from Divine Love flooded in. I found if I quieted my mind and paid attention, God/Goddess provided what I needed in each moment and more. This was one of Gary's last gifts—the recognition that Divine Spirit was my eternal partner, always walking right beside me. I felt Divine Love everywhere on my journey now.

The previous week, I had gone for a walk in the woods by the lake next to our house. I became aware of a loud moaning. It was the trees who were leaning against each other moving in the strong wind. Words appeared in my mind, *Lean on others in your grief, Robbie. You're not alone.*

Farther along the path was a tree that had grown in a fantastical crooked shape. Gary and I called it the "rhinoceros tree" because it looked for all the world like a giant rhinoceros with a horn. This time as I approached it, I noticed sap leaking out of the knot in the position of its "eye." The knot with sap leaking down looked distinctly like my rhinoceros was crying. Again words came into my mind, *God is crying with you.*

For a moment the message brought me comfort. Then I thought, *But how can I comfort God?*

A reply came almost immediately, *Comforting yourself will comfort Me.*

Every time I walked in the woods near our house during that week, I had a strong sense spiritual energy was intensifying around our property. It was as if the universe was converging its attention on Gary's passing. We seemed to have become a vortex of expectation.

One morning around five o'clock I stood at our picture window looking out at the lake. It was still dark and I saw a procession of car lights wrapping around the side of the lake. It was only the morning commuters making their way along the highway, but I'd never seen anything like it before. Their lights were reflecting on the surface of the lake as they moved along, reaching out in long brilliant lines. It was quite a sight—that procession of light.

Again, words appeared in my mind: *Many are coming in now for Gary's passing.*

I got a clear interpretation with those words: The beings in the Dreamtime—the celestial hosts from the universe that lies behind the universe—were gathering around us for Gary's passing.

I don't mean to sound egotistical for Gary about this. I think many people who have experienced a death or a birth have felt this whirlpool of spiritual energy around the event. Perhaps they have felt relatives who have crossed over were present. Or, maybe they have felt the presence of Divine Mother or angels or an ascended one like Jesus or the Buddha or the Prophet. For me, it was the first time I had been able to sense a spiritual gathering of this magnitude.

Many are coming in. Gathering on the other side of the veil, to welcome Gary and to comfort us.

On the evening of the day I had seen the lights on the lake, I walked up to the top of a saddle between two peaks on our mountain. I could feel the spiritual energy swirling there like a strong vortex, and I felt love pouring out from the trees and the rocks. I felt such gratitude and honor to have been part of this journey with Gary and to be so close to Divine Love. It was so humbling. As the tears rolled down my cheeks, I felt the breeze on the wetness there on my face.

I had a strong knowing that God was in this breeze. The breeze *was* God.

It took the tears of my grief to feel Divine Love with me in this moment.

The night after Gary lost consciousness, I had a vivid dream. I was trying to escape something and I took refuge in a roomful of angels. There were a number of us there, trying to hide among the angels, trying to blend in.

There was an angel with red curly hair to whom I was particularly drawn. "So how long you been an angel?" I asked him, just nonchalantly making conversation.

"Forever," he replied with a smile.

In the dream there was a ferry leaving, a barge that could take us humans to safety. You needed a ticket to get on this barge and fortunately I had mine in hand. As I was getting on, the person in front of me lost their ticket. I handed her mine. I knew I wouldn't be allowed to leave on the ferry and reach that place of safety (wherever that was), but I felt a surge of love for this stranger and had to help her.

It turned out the stranger was the red-haired angel's sister, and that selfless act would save me. As the barge was leaving, I ran down to the end of the dock, but the distance was too far to jump. I had an urge to jump anyway, and as I jumped the angels lifted me. I flew through the distance and landed safely on the barge.

It was a beautiful dream and I believe Spirit made sure I remembered it.

When I awoke the next morning, I was aware I had been in a room full of angels and that they were still there with Gary and me in his final days.

41

THE LAST PRECIOUS GIFTS

My last night with Gary before he passed, I lay tucked up next to him.

He appeared comatose, but I knew he was aware of me, because as I cuddled in beside him, with every ounce of strength he had left, he lifted his arm to hold me. I saw his signature white eye-shaped energy when I closed my eyes. I knew he was working on me, this time to send me increased love and ease my grief.

My heart was so open now, I saw love everywhere I looked: the freshly laundered folded clothes left outside our bedroom door by my sister, who didn't want to disturb us; my dog Checkers quietly waiting, ready to extend comfort the minute I stepped out; the beautiful yellow flowers that had been sent by a friend. God—Love—was everywhere around me and I was so aware of it in this heightened state of grief. In the last hours with Gary, those endless expressions of love were no longer taken for granted.

The last moments with Gary. Those are the gifts I cling to. The faint puff of his breath on my face. The squeeze of my hand returned by him, even in his deeply comatose state.

I knew I didn't have to speak out loud because he could always hear my thoughts. Like the Aborigines who rarely spoke out loud to each other while he was with them, we always enjoyed sitting in the silence together. But I did speak out loud. I kissed his head and said, "I love you."

It was almost inaudible. I barely heard him, but he did speak out loud. He said, "I love *you*. Thank you for being here." So I got my wish after all.

Later, I could feel his heart start to stutter and falter. The light energy coming from him was stronger than ever. As I washed his face, we had a moment of communion. I saw him seeing me with his psychic senses. I saw that he saw the energy of love pouring forth from me to him. I hadn't known it until that moment, but I realized he must always have seen the love coming from me, pouring out from me to him like a faithful wellspring. What a gift to know that.

How would I go on with my life after being with Gary? What could I do with my life that would be worthy of the gratitude I felt? What could I give him? I realized the best tribute to Gary I could make was to take good care of myself, to love myself fully—as he had quietly loved me. His care of me reminded me of Divine Mother's words given to me once by Karyn: "I will love you while you learn to love yourself." It was time to love myself.

I knew the message of Gary's life: *Don't wait until you have all your distractions taken away before you start talking to the Creator, the Source.* At what a high price that message had come. He wanted all of us to know: The best way to heal anything is trusting and giving your physical, emotional, and spiritual challenges over to God, *the healer within us.* The Divine One is where the healing really comes from, at a level of power unmatched by humankind.

I softly told him his lessons would not be wasted. "I will spend my life spreading these beautiful messages along with the others."

The next morning, something was different and the animals sensed it.

My dog, Checkers, refused to eat his breakfast—something he had never done before. Even though Checkers was my most devoted companion and almost never left my side, this morning he went and quietly lay down in his own bed in the kitchen and wouldn't get up. He seemed to have a deep sadness.

Peeps, the male cockatiel, sang his parting song, the song he always sang to his babies when they were leaving. He sang for about half an hour. I like to think he sang to Gary about where he was going and how much he would be loved there.

Buns, our female cockatiel, had been laying a clutch for several days. She laid the last egg that morning. It was the only egg she ever laid that didn't hatch.

I rarely left Gary's side in those last final hours, but that morning an old friend stopped by about ten o'clock. It was one of Gary's previous caregivers, Charlene, a beautiful woman from Belize with a heart of gold contained in a petite little body. Charlene wanted to see how Gary was doing. I left Gary for a few minutes while Charlene, my sister Lynn, and I talked briefly in the kitchen.

When I returned to Gary's side a few minutes later, I discovered he had passed. He slipped away in the few minutes I was gone. I'm sure he knew it would be easier for me to be out of the room in the moment of his final breath.

I tearfully rejoined my sister and Charlene in the kitchen and relayed that Gary had just peacefully passed to the other side.

As we all embraced each other and cried, my sister noticed that right outside the kitchen window on our deck lay a dead hummingbird. It was the little hummingbird who had watched me all week as I sat at the kitchen table.

42

FINALLY DANCING

As I moved through the intense grief of physically losing Gary, I felt despair and pain more profound than I ever imagined could exist, something you can never truly know until you've been to the deepest place of pain within. But Gary taught me well. I asked and allowed Divine Oneness to comfort me.

What I did not anticipate was still feeling Gary so strongly. I could see Gary's light, the unique eye-shaped light behind my eyelids. I was seeing that light of healing love, and it was brighter than ever before.

The moment I became aware in the mornings, before I had opened my eyes, he was there. When I meditated, his light of love was there waiting for me. When I closed my eyes and called to him throughout the day, within minutes the light appeared and I could feel his presence.

I went about my days, but I didn't want to forget the new wisdom I had gained from the heavy price of losing Gary. I wanted to remember to slow down my body and my busy mind. I wanted to take the time to see and feel what was really valuable in life: the subtle gifts of love, comfort, strength, and guidance Divine Love was always sending.

I had another reason to slow down and feel within—another reason to quiet my mind and let my soul breathe—and that was to feel Gary as he spoke to me from the other side.

The day after Gary died I was listening to our courtship song, "Surrender" by Josh Groban. It's a song about feeling yourself surrender, feeling your heart fall into place. It perfectly expressed what I felt when I fell in love with Gary.

I was standing there, swaying to the music with my eyes closed. Tears ran down my cheeks and dripped from my chin. I just let them.

Then I heard a message in my mind. Very clear. *Calm down . . . relax . . . stop crying . . . just dance.*

I felt Gary. It was like his arms were around me and I found myself dancing steps I didn't know how to dance. He was leading me. It was something like a tango with lots of turns and swirls in place. The light of his presence was bright behind my closed eyes. We were dancing— this was the day I discovered what a beautiful dancer Gary had been in his lifetime.

Immediately after Gary died, my family flew out from the Midwest. You couldn't have kept them away. They were wonderful in every way.

They helped me host a memorial at my house that I called, "A Celebration of Gary's Life." We put up banners and Hawaiian leis and had little displays all about the house. One banner said, "Welcome Home." Another said, "Till We Meet Again."

Gary's body had been cremated and I had some of the ashes placed into a platinum gold heart. Gary's favorite expression is engraved across the top: "Love is All."

I also had some of his ashes placed inside a cup sealed onto a delicate wind chime. It contributed lovely soft musical tones all afternoon as spring breezes wafted through the house and guests passed by.

The memorial was on a beautiful sunny spring day and there were hummingbirds everywhere, buzzing the guests on the deck. Many people commented about it, saying they had never seen so many hummingbirds in one place. It was obvious the little warriors weren't going to be left out of the celebration.

Of course dozens of friends were there, including our friend Karyn, who channeled Divine Mother for us and could see into other dimensions. At the end of the celebration, she told me she had spent the entire afternoon watching Gary as he was living now on the other side of the veil. "He was dancing around with the angels and Divine Mother and all his Aboriginal buddies, just enjoying all the stories people were telling about him. He was so excited and happy." I thanked her for telling me.

At the end of the celebration, some of us went out in a small boat to scatter Gary's ashes on the lake. I scattered red rose petals on the water along with the ashes. The roses made a beautiful sight floating away over the white boat's reflection in the sunlight.

I had chosen a song to be played during the momentous event of spreading Gary's ashes. As I began to strew the rose petals, I told my son Colin to go down into the wheelhouse and turn on the CD player. I had put a lot of forethought into picking this particular song and had it carefully cued up. Colin only needed to push "Play." But when Colin pushed the button, it was another song entirely that played!

Instead of the song I had set up, what played was "You Raise Me Up."

I listened as Josh Groban sang about being troubled and sitting still and waiting in the silence until "you come and sit awhile with me." About being raised up to stand on mountains and to walk on stormy seas. And about glimpsing eternity in each other.

Thanks, Gary.

43
STILL A TEAM

I looked around the room and saw that once again they had run out of places to sit. The class was taking place at a food co-op in a nearby town. The organizers were busy setting up more chairs in the back of the room for the people who continued to pour in.

The time to begin the class arrived and the happy chatter quieted down. The audience sat with pens poised over their notepads, waiting for me to start.

I opened my mouth, but I couldn't speak.

It wasn't stage fright keeping me frozen. I was afraid that if I made any sound, I would burst into tears.

This was the first class I was teaching without Gary.

The class, titled "Aboriginal Healing Secrets," had been on my calendar for months. It had been scheduled for a day only two weeks after Gary died. Friends encouraged me to cancel. But I had a strong feeling I should go ahead, that Gary wanted me to teach it. My friends said I was in denial.

Since I started speaking six years ago, I had never been at a loss for words in any teaching situation . . . until today. Oh man, had my friends been right?

What had I been thinking coming here?

I had lost my soul mate only two weeks ago. I was still stumbling around in a zombie state, tissues stuffed in my pockets ready for a sudden onset of tears at any moment. During the days leading up to tonight, I could barely say Gary's name out loud, let alone describe his journey into the Outback to a roomful of people.

I had thought about canceling. When I imagined teaching this two-hour class, I couldn't see how I would have the emotional strength to pull it off. It was too close to home. This was his story and his teachings. Every word I spoke would ooze Gary's energy and bring vividly back to me memories of him and our time together.

I had anguished over whether to cancel the class. I wanted to listen to my heart's direction and not my frightened mind with its dire predictions of failure and embarrassment. In the end I decided to go ahead and teach the class, knowing that was what Gary would want.

Where was the strength I had counted on? My confidence was draining as if from a sieve. I felt sure I was going to break down.

I thought of sending them all home and rescheduling, but I was afraid I would start crying even as I explained to the room why we had to cancel. At the moment, I was still calm on the outside, but inside I couldn't seem to pull it together and either start the class or cancel it.

This was such a bad idea. Of course you should have canceled this. What were you thinking, Robbie?! The internal beatings were still so quick to start up.

Other than a woman in the back sifting through her purse, the packed room was absolutely still. The attendees patiently waited for me to begin, their expectant eyes resting on me with detached interest. No one there knew what I was going through.

I felt like I was going to be sick to my stomach.

I prayed, *Gary, please give me the strength to do this. Help me, sweetheart!* I took a deep breath and nervously smiled at the roomful of faces.

"Hi, I'm Robbie Holz," I said. "Thank you for joining me tonight."

It was subtle at first, but I could discern a loving energy flowing into my trembling body. As I relaxed a little more, I could detect this loving force increasing in strength. It built throughout the evening. It seemed to flow into me, but also to swirl in the air around me, so that I felt held—supported in it like fruit in Jell-O, only warmer. I was shocked that I was not only able to open my mouth, I didn't falter once throughout my presentation. The participants would never have known I had lost the love of my life only two weeks ago.

Just like when he was alive, Gary had not failed me. He had pumped me up and given me strength. Even from the other dimension, Gary helped me. I kept going strong throughout the entire two-hour presentation.

When the last attendee left the classroom, I grabbed the rest room keys and quickly walked to the ladies room. It was the type that was meant for one person at a time. Unlocking the old wooden door, I had barely stepped inside when I burst uncontrollably into tears. "Thank you, baby," I said aloud.

I slid to the blue-tiled floor and sat there in my skirt in a crumbled heap and wept. "How am I going to do this without you, love? I miss you so much." I cried for a long time and felt layers of grief release from my petite body.

I slowly got up and smoothed out my skirt with my hands, grateful no one had wanted to use the bathroom. Walking over to the sink, I splashed cold water on my face. Looking in the mirror at my red and swollen eyes, normally my critical mind would have been judgmental. Instead I felt pride and kindness swelling in my heart.

"We did it. Looks like we're still a team, sweetie."

44

A SECOND WOOING

At first, to seek out being with Gary was too painful. To have encounters with his spirit was a beautiful gift, but it was just too much for my broken heart to bear. I wasn't ready to see him in my dreams. I wasn't ready to hear him speak to me in my mind. My grief was so intense I would cry when the wind chime gently tinkled, or when a paper on which I had—inexplicably—written, "Love you, babe," fluttered to the floor at my feet.

My poor, hurting, human self drew away from anything that would kindle that pain.

In a way, Gary had to woo me all over again.

We had a rather unique set of friends, Gary and I. Some of them were seers who could communicate with the other side, and Gary would appear to them and send me messages, just as he had asked Martha to call me with his job offer so many years ago. I got calls from our friends saying Gary was helping them in their healing work, had appeared to them in a dream, or had just showed up with a message for me. Usually, the message was, *I'm so proud of you.*

Sometimes he showed up to give them advice on their cooking.

This happened with Meredith. Meredith was Gary's longtime psychic friend whom Gary had taken house hunting in order to be sure his soul mate—me—would love the house he bought. One day she left a message for me on my answering machine.

"I just had to call and tell you what happened to me last night," Meredith told me in her usual cheery, straightforward way. "You'll get a kick out of this. I'm in the kitchen cooking and Gary shows up in some kind of '70s outfit. You know the bell-bottom pants? Not unfashionable, but looking really good—he looked gorgeous—very young and ageless and so happy. I've seen people who have passed before, so he knows I'm not alarmed. He walks over to the stove, leans over and takes a whiff of the vegetable stew I've got cooking on the stove for the boys. 'You're gonna need some onion in that,' he tells me. 'Yeah, I'm thinking about it,' I told him. 'Really,' he tells me, 'it'll make a difference.' I'm getting a little testy about someone telling me how to cook, so I told him, 'I know, I know, I'm getting around to it.'" The message machine recorded her laughter. Then she continued, "So I put the damn onion in it. And I'll be darned, he was right, it needed onion."

She was still laughing when she hung up and the recording ended.

Even though it made me cry when I first heard it, I played the message over and over. I had only ever known Gary as a paraplegic in a wheelchair. It felt so good to hear how he had "walked over" to the stove, how he was dressed as he had been in his twenties, how he was young and happy. I left that phone message on my machine for months and played it whenever I needed to hear words that would bring comfort to my heart.

For a year after he passed, I got e-mails and phone calls all conveying the same messages: *Gary is happy. He's there for you whenever you need him. He's so proud of you.*

Sometimes I would get a message from a complete stranger. Like the time I was taking a class and a woman I had only just met—who knew nothing of my history—came up to me. "Excuse me, this may sound really strange," she said.

"I doubt it," I replied.

She continued sheepishly and a bit bewildered, "Well, there's this guy I'm seeing in my mind's eye. He's got a beard and he's dancing around. He clearly wants me to convey . . . he's dancing around and jumping up and down . . . I know this sounds crazy, but he wants me to tell you he loves the freedom of not being in his physical body. Does that make sense to you?"

"Perfectly. Thank you," I said, and walked away smiling.

A few months after Gary passed, I went to a summer festival in Oregon celebrating Mother Earth. A couple hundred people came from all over the world. We were camped in a mountain meadow, sheltered all around by trees. At night we came together and sang around a bonfire, sending gratitude to our beautiful planet.

On the last night, a dozen of us diehards were still around the bonfire. Someone was playing the violin. It was cold, and I saw a tall, slender old man with a gray beard standing with a blanket wrapped around him. Despite the blanket, I could see he was shivering in the night air. He was quite elderly. Being friendly, I went up to this old man to help warm him up. I cozied up inside the blanket against his stomach with my back to him. He wrapped his arms around me as we stood together singing.

Suddenly it became clear to me that Gary was there. Even though I was being held by the elderly man, Gary was holding me through the old man's body. At around six feet tall, the old guy was about the same height as Gary and his soft, gray beard against the top of my head felt like Gary's beard.

I got such a strong distinct feeling that Gary was coming through this old man whose arms were wrapped around me that I started quietly crying. I felt tears flowing down my cheeks.

No one seemed to notice my tears in the darkness. I unashamedly accepted this beautiful gift—to have Gary's presence comforting me through this old man. Over the months I had come to accept that Gary was with me in spirit and in my thoughts, but I missed him so much physically. I allowed myself to be held for just this few minutes.

The next day I asked the elderly man if he had minded my breaking down like that, and he said, "Didn't bother me a bit. I don't know what it was all about, but I thought it was great!"

A month or so after the festival, I had a dream from Gary. He was with me on a beach. At first I didn't recognize him, but then I looked into his incredibly beautiful light-blue eyes with the gold flecks and knew that I was looking at his soul. An overpowering longing for him rose up in me. At one point in the dream, he was able to hold me, standing behind me just as the old man at the bonfire had.

It was a brief touch, but I woke with gratitude that I had been able to spend time with him in a dream. I knew then that I was healing, because in the morning I felt joyful, instead of crying for hours as I had before when I had had dreams about him. It had been too painful then, but now I welcomed it.

45

ACCEPTING LOVE

Eventually, I began to read books about the afterlife, absorbing the ideas that felt like truth to me. I had so many questions.

Where had he gone? What was he doing? What greeted him when he initially passed out of his body? Was he off working? Learning? Would I be keeping him from more important things by calling him to me? Could he hear me at all?

Over time I discovered that the rules of time and space don't apply in the Dreamtime. Gary was (is) able to be in many places at the same time. And he was more than happy to come to me, or anyone else who needed him.

Every morning at 8:00 I saw Gary's healing light—the characteristic eye-shaped light on the inside of my eyes when I closed them. Not at 7:59. Not at 8:01. As punctual as Gary was in life, he was equally punctual reaching through from the other side.

That tradition continues to this day. He shows up to spend time with me at 8:00 a.m. The only time he missed the appointment was the first time Daylight Saving Time switched in the spring. (In most of the United States we set our clocks back an hour on an agreed upon day in the fall and forward an hour on another day in the spring.) Gary missed it. He was an hour late. I teased him about that. He never made that mistake again.

I became more and more comfortable with having Gary be present in my life.

I began communicating with him intentionally. I started using Gary's wedding ring on the end of some embroidery floss as a pendulum. (The use of a pendulum to get answers from the other side is a very old tradition.) Sometimes I would ask him, "Are you still madly in love with me?" and his ring would swing wildly backward and forward—the answer for *Yes!*

He loved to use songs to communicate with me. Often a song would suddenly pop into my head, and when I realized how appropriate it was for what I was feeling, I knew it was Gary. For example, he would send Stevie Wonder's "Don't You Worry 'Bout a Thing" if I was feeling anxious and scared. Or Bette Midler's "Wind Beneath My Wings" if I was low and depressed. That was his way of telling me he was always there, lifting me up. Sometimes if my mind was so busy spinning around my worries that I couldn't hear a song in my head, he would arrange for the perfect song to actually play on the radio.

I had a little altar on my bedroom dresser. The display had an image for Divine Mother and other places I had experienced the presence of the Divine. I would light candles or incense and use it to aid my meditation and my intentioning. If I had something I wanted—more inner peace, or a trip to swim with dolphins—I would put it in a special box on my little altar. It was my focal point. I wanted Gary near, so I added Gary's picture to the display and the platinum heart that contained some of his ashes, which read: "Love is All." I also added other things of his that I put in a colorful bowl Gary had given me. In the glaze of the bowl were words that read: "What lies behind us and before us are tiny matters compared to what lies within us."

And then there were the red roses.

After Gary passed, I missed him the most on his birthday, Valentine's Day, and the anniversary of his death. On those dates I would place a red rose for him next to his picture. Gary used to find all sorts of surprising ways to get me a red rose on those same days. I would open my mail and find an advertisement with a red rose featured prominently. Or one of my friends would "just happen" to send me a newsletter with a red rose image. One Valentine's Day I went out to dinner with a girlfriend. At the end of the meal, the waiter gave us each a red rose. Every time one of those days came around, I could expect Gary to come up with an imaginative method of getting me a rose. He was ever the romantic.

Another time, I went to a service at a local church to pass out brochures for a charity I work with (Heroes for the Homeless, if you're looking for a good one). It just happened to be the Memorial Day weekend, and to my surprise, the focus of the service was honoring the continuing relationship we have with our loved ones who have crossed over.

As the congregation sang "May the circle be unbroken . . ." people moved to the altar and placed flowers for their departed loved ones there. It was so moving to see the flowers increasing into great mounds—so much love continuing on, reaching across the divide. There was every kind of flower imaginable.

Because I hadn't known about the tradition in this church, I hadn't brought any flowers to place on the altar. Suddenly, a woman in front of me turned around and gave me one of hers. A red rose. I placed it on the altar next to some Stargazer Lilies, which were always Gary's favorites.

Mostly, to feel Gary I merely started paying attention. A puff of breeze on my cheek as I was sitting on our special bench under the trees, or a birdcall at exactly the right moment—these were little things that surrounded me throughout my day and said, "Hi babe, I'm still here. I still love you."

How did I know it was Gary?

You can only push the coincidence theory so far. The little signs were too synchronistic. Often some small thing would happen to interrupt me if I was thoughtlessly doing something that wasn't good for me. The potato chip bag would fall out of my hand. Or a limb would clunk against the roof when my thoughts strayed into fearful territory.

It didn't take much to see that there was an intelligence and love behind these interruptions.

But most of all, I could *feel* it. I could feel it because Gary had taught me how to feel and see Divine Love when it manifested.

Like the Aborigines, Gary sensed that everything made by the Big Guy is love. And it's everywhere. It's everywhere and everything. "Love is All." It's the air we breathe and the water we drink. A tree is an expression of Divine Love in the form of a tree. Even we, in all our supposed imperfection and with all our limitations, we are made of love. Gary had taught me how to feel and see this divine energy of love and life.

Several months after Gary passed, I realized that I hadn't had a vacation away from home in a long, long time. So I decided to take a break and go to the beach. I stayed in a yurt by the ocean in Oregon. I deliberately set the intention, "I'm going on vacation with Gary and with God/Goddess." If you get to choose your travel companions, you might as well choose the best.

At one point I was sitting on top of a sandy hill overlooking the ocean. It was a gorgeous, brisk day. I was nestled down in the beach grasses that divided the inland area from the beach, and all sorts of people were playing down below on the sand. Families were flying kites, building sand castles, and having picnics. Couples were walking hand in hand, letting the waves kick up around their ankles.

I sat watching them, taking it all in, feeling warm and slightly detached. When the sun started to set, people packed up their gear and funneled back to their cars by walking between two dunes, one of which I was sitting on. It was as if they were in a procession as they walked back to their cars with the setting sun behind them.

With no warning, I suddenly felt the strongest wave of love go through my body that I had ever experienced. I felt such incredible love for them, way beyond anything a human being could feel for strangers leaving a beach. This wave of love came with a clear and certain inner knowing: I was feeling the smallest fraction of the love the Divine has for us. By letting me feel just a little bit of the Divine's love for these strangers, I was being shown how truly loved we are. I knew it was a gift from Gary and Divine Love.

I decided in that moment to spend my life helping people as much as I am able. I took a picture of where I was sitting on top of the sandy hill overlooking the ocean. That picture is on my altar. It's a reminder to me of how much we are loved—that we aren't capable of grasping even a tiny fraction of the love that is given to us.

About a year after Gary passed, I noticed as I sat quietly eating my meals, there was a little hummingbird who always seemed to be joining me. It would sit on the same spot the other hummingbird had, perched on the top branch of the white-flowering tree. The tree had just started to sprout its new spring buds.

Gary may have been just a spirit without a physical body, but I invited him to my meals and we sat quietly together enjoying each others' company—Gary in spirit, the hummingbird outside, and me.

46

MY CHECKER-HELPING MIND

"Checkers! Come here. Come on." I patted the top of my thigh, calling Checkers back to me and my sister on the trail.

Lynn and I were taking our two dogs on the usual route through the woods. Lynn had recently started looking for work. She would be moving out soon and I would be alone in my Keyserville house above the lake. All alone with my memories in that enormous house. The prospect loomed like a gaping hole in my future. Yet I knew Lynn needed to move on with her life—and soon.

Uncharacteristically, Checkers ignored me. He took off up the hill through the thick underbrush. Chasing the fresh scent of squirrel perhaps?

I hollered, "Checkers come!" in the clearly commanding voice to which Checkers normally responded. (We'd had a lot of dog training classes.) But he didn't listen. Undeterred, he was now out of sight. I could hear him thrashing in the bushes even farther off the path.

"Checkers, get over here! Now!" I yelled at him. I had quickly gone beyond commanding and into furious.

The only response was more rustling, getting fainter. "Checkers COME! Damn it!"

Lynn winced and gave me a quick look, but she didn't say anything.

Her dog, Tex, darted back to us from up the path, as if to say, *Hey, at least I'm a good boy.*

Hearing the anger in my voice, Checkers abandoned his instinctive desire to chase squirrels and obediently returned to my side.

"Good boy." I grudgingly gave him a pat on the head and grimaced at his fur, which was now tangled with bits of bramble, thistle, and dead leaves. I didn't look at my sister. Guilt had set in. I had ruined the mood of our nice walk.

Our childhood family hated confrontation. Consequently, we were all very sensitive to raised voices and angry words. Cursing was not something that had ever been done in our house. It took a lot to get me angry, especially at an animal, but my temper had been increasingly quick to surface lately, and we both knew it. As we continued the walk, I could feel my sister darting concerned glances my way.

Finally, I flashed her an apologetic look. "Sorry I lost my temper."

"It's all right," Lynn said. The sympathy in her voice made me feel even worse. "I know you're under a lot of pressure right now."

Lynn knew me well and she had felt the mounting tension. Since the beginning of the summer, I had been struggling. In my heart I knew it was time to sell the house that she and Gary and I had shared. However, I was strongly resisting the message. Actually, I was completely rejecting it.

Our house held all the memories of my life with Gary. I felt if I left the house, I was going to lose more of him. Pieces of our memories were lodged in every room. I was afraid that if the house went, my memories of our times together would fade and go as well. The house was like a security blanket. I was hanging on to it for every ounce of comfort it could provide. I was clinging to my security blanket/house . . . despite the mounting signs that it was time to leave.

It was the fall of 2007, only five months since Gary's passing. But the housing bubble had burst. There was talk of banks failing. Unemployment was soaring. Economists were predicting a depression worse than the Great Depression of the 1930s. There was financial fear everywhere. Everyone who cared about me kept telling me to put my house up for sale and get out—now.

"You're right," I said. "I feel the pressure to sell the house before the housing market gets any worse." I shook my head. "I hear what they're saying. I just can't part with the one place Gary and I shared our . . ." My voice trailed off. I couldn't say it out loud. . . . *our life together. Our physical life together that was over now.*

"Well, Gary is still looking out for you," Lynn reminded me. "He won't leave you, just because you leave the house."

"I know he wouldn't. I know he won't abandon me wherever I go. I know it in my head, but my heart is still aching. I want to hold on to something physical. I guess I'm afraid I'll lose even more of him if I move away . . . and I'm not sure I can bear to lose anything else."

I tossed a long stick down the path for the dogs and we watched them retrieve it together, both holding on to an end—the branch manager and the assistant branch manager.

"Ask for help from your team," my sister suggested.

"I have been. I keep handing the situation over to Divine Mother, Gary, and the rest of my celestial team." I laughed ruefully. "Apparently, I keep bungee-cording it back to me because my mind keeps trying to figure out an alternate solution. Even though I know my mind is just 'Checker helping.' It's not coming up with anything useful, but it's sure busy trying."

"Those financial worries," Lynn agreed, shaking her head. "They're tough. They can be Super Glued on . . . if we're too attached to the outcome. You know . . . if the solution has to look a certain way."

"You're right. I know what my team is telling me to do, but I don't like where their guidance is leading me."

We slipped into silence as we walked along the path under the gray Northwest sky.

"I know my spiritual team has great things in store for me and that I have to let go of the house to move on to them. If I keep resisting, I see myself getting more and more isolated, holing up on my acreage in the boonies. They know what's best for me, but . . . I'm still afraid." I paused. "I can feel the fear draining my energy and pulling me down. I've got insomnia again. And the darn junk food . . . I don't want to get sick again."

"You don't want to get sick again," Lynn agreed.

"I know Gary cleared the last of the hep C right out of my body. I haven't tested positive for it for years. But when I get really energetically depleted like this, I get scared it might come back." My voice sounded small and frail to my ears.

My sister reached over and gave my back a vigorous rub. "You know Gary is still there working for you—your whole team is—they can handle whatever you give them. It's easy for them. They can *do* it."

Suddenly Lynn stopped in the path and flapped her arms in a precision cheerleading routine that immediately cracked me up. She ended with a fairly impressive vertical stag leap, swooping her imaginary pom-poms high into the air.

"Go-oooooo Team!"

I paused in the middle of the path and spread my arms open to the sky. With confused looks on their faces, both dogs were stopped in their tracks watching these two women: *What the heck are they doing now?*

"I surrender my finances, career, and health to my team—again!" I laughed out loud.

I paused. Darn it. I could still feel a persistent fear wrapped around my heart, refusing to completely let go. "Help guide me to abundance, a fulfilling career, and happiness," I followed up.

"Can I piggyback on that?" Lynn asked, smiling.

"Of course!" I said.

On our return climb up the hill to the house, I watched Checkers cavorting around us and wondered what it would take for my team to loosen my controlling mind's tight grip.

Help me get my mind out of the way and follow your guidance, I prayed. . . . *In an easy, gentle, grace-filled way,* I quickly added.

47

AN APARTMENT

As Lynn and I pulled up to the two-story house with a "For Rent" sign in the front yard, my former husband Aaron and his girlfriend Mindy waved us to an available parking spot. When Lynn and I got out of the car, there were warm hugs all around.

"Thank you so much for calling us," I said. "Lynn's been looking for a place for weeks. I can't believe we were only a few minutes away from here when you called."

Lynn and I were still living in the house outside of Keyserville. It was the spring of 2008 and Lynn had started a new job. Unfortunately, her job was an hour-and-a-half commute from Keyserville. This place was five minutes away from her new job. If we had been at home this morning, it would have been an hour-and-a-half drive to check out this apartment. Aaron had caught us while we were running an errand only minutes away.

"Good thing we went this way," Aaron said. "We normally don't go down this block on our morning walk."

Aaron and I had been divorced for more than eight years. Our relationship had settled into a cherished friendship, the kind of rare friendship you can have only with someone when you also share a wonderful son and thirty years of common memories. Separately, we had both

211

gotten to a place where we knew we had made the right decision to split up. Aaron was the first person to call me after Gary died, offering his compassion and assistance. I was so grateful to have this honorable, loving man still in my life.

"How'd you even know I was looking?" Lynn asked, bewildered. She had taken her new job two months ago and had no luck finding an apartment that was both nearby and affordable.

"Colin told me about an hour ago. He came by looking to borrow an extra life jacket for a spur-of-the-moment canoe trip this afternoon."

"Well, thanks for looking out for us," I said.

Aaron and Mindy led the way down a dirt path lined with daffodils to the carriage-house-style apartment behind the main house. "We checked it out through the window," Mindy said. "It's really cute."

Aaron lived in Richards, a little town north of Seattle perched in a bowl of land centered above a ferry landing. The town was quaint, safe, and had a friendly community feeling—a town where the locals all say "Hi" to one another as they walk the waterfront promenade. This place was in a great neighborhood of Richards—quiet, surrounded by parks, and only a couple blocks from the water and the lovely snow-topped mountain views.

It was spring and the small yard was filled with fragrant flowering trees and bushes. A gigantic white tulip tree was in full bloom, and a stunning pink-blossomed magnolia stretched up to the second-story apartment.

"It's cool, isn't it?" Aaron said, as he pointed to the apartment at the top of the stairs.

"Oh my gosh, it's beautiful." Lynn put her hand to her mouth.

Lynn and I climbed the wooden stairs, which were tastefully painted in a vaguely nautical navy, white, and burgundy.

We had just reached the landing when suddenly a hummingbird appeared out of nowhere and buzzed us both in the face, one after the other. We both jumped, startled. It was the first hummingbird we had seen this year.

"What was that about?" Lynn cried out. But it was only rhetorical. Without even entering the apartment, we both knew her search was over—this was to be her new home. Gary was making that very clear.

We peeked through a window into the empty apartment. It was spotless inside with sleek hardwood floors and elegant black handles on the kitchen cabinets.

"We're gonna head out," Aaron called out from below. "Hope it works out for you."

With my hands placed across my heart, I said, "Thank you so much."

"Thanks. I really appreciate it," Lynn called after them as they resumed their morning walk.

She pulled out her cell phone and dialed the number posted on the sign. After a quick conversation, she hung up and turned to me with an amused look. "The realtor said her dental appointment was unexpectedly canceled, so she'll be here in a few minutes."

Less than five minutes later, the rental manager showed up, a middle-aged brunette, all smiles. As she fumbled with finding the right key, she commented, "I only put up the sign a few hours ago, and I already have a young woman who has paid a deposit. Looks like she's going to rent it, but I'll be happy to show it to you anyway."

"It's already rented?" Lynn was completely shocked.

That's not right, I thought. *That's got to be a mistake.*

"She's first in line, but you're welcome to fill out an application and give me a deposit for a background check in case she doesn't take it."

Lynn was clearly deflated. It only took a few minutes to go through the modest one-bedroom apartment. It had recently been remodeled. Lynn and I fell in love with the cozy place immediately. It was perfect.

I expected Lynn to pull out her checkbook to put down a deposit. But instead, she said, "I'll think about it and let you know in a few days."

"Lynn," I said. "Can I talk to you for a second?"

"I'll be just outside," the manager said and discreetly stepped out.

I closed the front door behind the realtor, who started to pull off wilted flowers on the bush overhanging the landing.

"Aren't you going to put down a deposit and get your name second on the list?" I asked.

"I want to sleep on it before I do anything."

"Lynn, if you wait a day longer, the list of people wanting to rent this place will be a mile long." She was going to let this amazing gift slip through her fingers. I couldn't believe it.

"Well, somebody's already got it. What's the point?" Lynn argued.

"This place is supposed to be yours! Look at all the synchronicities it took to get us here." I started ticking off my fingers. "Colin just happens to tell Aaron an hour ago that you're looking for a place. Aaron just happens to take a different route on his morning walk. The sign just happens to have gone up only a few hours ago. We just happen to be here in Richards when we get the call. The property manager just happens to have had her dental appointment canceled, so she's available to take your deposit—"

"And someone else just happens to have rented it before we got here," Lynn cut me off.

"We both got buzzed by a hummingbird, for God's sake. You know who that's a sign from," I countered.

"Yeah, I know," Lynn replied. But she was still unconvinced. "I just want to sleep on it before I do anything. I don't like giving her my money when someone else already has the place."

"Look, you know Gary loves you and is clearly looking out for you. He and your spiritual team led you to this place because they're taking care of you. You've been asking for help—now accept it." I understood her reticence. This was advice I'd given myself time and time again, and quite recently. For some reason, our ego-mind just doesn't want to give anyone else a turn at the steering wheel.

"All right," Lynn said, reluctantly. "I'd still prefer to sleep on it, but I'll put down the deposit and fill out the application."

"Good!"

"But I'm gonna keep looking."

"Fine. But you know you're going to get this place."

I breathed a sigh of relief. Then, immediately I felt a twinge of sadness. Lynn was going to be moving out of the home we'd shared for the past three years. It was going to be completely empty. How would I ever endure it once she left?

The following Saturday, Lynn left our house early in the morning to look for another apartment. Around noon she called me and I immediately heard the frustration in her voice.

"I had six appointments scheduled today to view apartments. Every single appointment canceled on me. Six of 'em! I don't know what's going on."

"I do," I said, perhaps a bit smugly.

"Well, then please enlighten me," Lynn wailed.

"You're not supposed to get any of those places. Don't you get it? You're supposed to get that cute place over the carriage house in Richards."

"No, *you* don't get it. That place is already rented. Remember?" Lynn sounded annoyed.

"I know it looks that way to you, but there are too many obvious signs that keep pointing to the carriage-house apartment. You think it's a coincidence that today all six of your appointments fell through? You know you're going to love what your team has picked out for you—unless you get nervous and settle for less."

"Well, then I'm going to start asking for more trust and patience, because my mind is going crazy." Lynn sighed, then said reluctantly, "Thanks, I guess I feel a little better."

A few days later, as I was sitting down to a lunch of tomato soup, the phone rang.

"You won't believe what just happened." It was Lynn and she sounded excited.

"Tell me."

"You know that place above the carriage house that you were so sure was supposed to be mine but it was already rented?" There was a brief hesitation, then Lynn burst out, "It's mine!"

I laughed out loud. "Of course it is. Tell me what happened."

"The realtor just called to say I can have it if I want it. The young gal who was supposed to get it didn't make it through the credit check. I can move in whenever I want."

"Congratulations! I'm thrilled for you. You're going to love it there."

"I gotta go. I'm on my lunch hour but I wanted you to know right away. Love you. Bye," and she was gone.

"Love you too," I said to the empty phone and was surprised to find myself holding back tears. I was genuinely happy for Lynn. She deserved the best. With the new place a few minutes from her new job, she'd no longer have to endure the grueling over-three-hours-for-the-round-trip commute to work.

And I could feel cold fear already settling into my chest. Lynn hadn't moved out yet but I was already missing her. We adored each other and I loved having her around—we always had so much fun together. I was immensely grateful she had continued to live with me and keep me company for an entire year after Gary died. But Lynn had her own life now that involved a new job an hour and a half away. Now she couldn't be a buffer to the loneliness, the void that occupied my heart since Gary died.

Less than two weeks later, ten friends, Lynn, and I were loading Lynn's possessions into a small truck in the clear early-morning air.

"I'll follow the truck and meet you there," I yelled to Lynn as the truck pulled away. I slid behind the steering wheel of my car, which was filled with Lynn's fragile items: living room lamps, treasured framed pictures, and kitchen glassware. Like a caravan, we all started down my long driveway canopied under tall evergreens.

We pulled on to the road and headed for the main highway. I was directly behind Lynn as we pulled onto the bridge that signaled she was leaving our island. I would have thought a swarm of hummingbirds might escort Lynn over the bridge to her new home, but Divine Love decided to do it up right.

Just as Lynn and her truck were in the center of the bridge length, a bald eagle suddenly appeared. With its impressive seven-foot wingspan, it rode the wind directly over Lynn's truck, escorting her across the bridge to her new life. From my vantage point driving behind her, I watched in awe.

"You are the wind beneath my wings . . ."

"Nice touch, team," I said out loud. "I know she's in good hands."

48

PREPARING FOR AUSTRALIA

In June of 2008, my new friend, John Mendel, was pacing my living room floor and speaking on the phone to his friends in Australia: "Yes, she's teaching healing principles that her husband learned from the Jaripuyjangu when he stayed with them in their settlement. He had MS and they helped him . . . uh-huh . . . She's working on finishing and publishing his book . . . right, great. I'll get you her e-mail and you can work out the details." He snapped the phone shut and turned to me. "It's all set. You can stay with Angela and Quinton for a week before meeting with the Aboriginal women for the ceremonies."

"John, I'm not sure that I'll be able to do this. I have to arrange the financing—"

"Robbie, you know you have to go. Right?"

He *was* right. I knew I needed to go on this trip the day I received the invitation to join the group—a group of twenty white women invited by the Jaripuyjangu tribe to participate in a weeklong set of women's ceremonies at a sacred site near the great sandstone monolith, Uluru. It was an incredible honor to be invited.

John was a remarkable and deeply spiritual man. His passion was creating a better world with sustainable eco-friendly farming practices. As an importer of fair-trade coffee beans, his job allowed him to travel to many foreign places. He had contacts with indigenous people all over the world.

He had been instrumental in getting me the invitation to the Australian Aborigines' ceremonies and had shown up today because, instinctively, he had known I was hesitating about booking the trip. By the time he left my house, he had arranged everything: my schedule, where I would stay and with whom, and transportation from place to place. He had even initiated contact with locals who could arrange some speaking events for me while I was in Australia.

I had met John some months before through mutual friends. Gradually, I became aware that he hoped a romance might bloom between us. I had instantly put that idea out of my mind. It was only a year and some months since Gary had died, and I was still struggling for a vision of my life without him. How was I going to carry on our work? What did it mean to have Gary present in his spiritual form in my life? How could I ever consider another romantic interest? I couldn't. I was still married, even though my husband no longer had a physical body.

When I received the invitation to join this very special collaboration with the Jaripuyjangu women, I immediately knew that I should go on the trip. And I also immediately knew that it was, of course, impossible—financially and logistically.

So, I handed it over to my celestial team. *Okay, Divine Mother, Aboriginal friends, Gary, guides and angels, if you want this to happen, help me come up with the financing and help me make the arrangements.*

I'm not sure I really believed they would—but in September of 2008, I was on a plane bound for Australia. Let that be a lesson. Didn't someone once say, "Be careful what you wish for . . ."

Not only was I on my way, but my good friend Karyn—the woman who had channeled messages to Gary and me from Divine Mother for so many years—was with me.

When I told Karyn that I believed she should come to the Outback of Australia with me, she had thought it highly amusing. Not a chance! She was hardly a world traveler. And if she was going to start traveling the world, she wouldn't start with camping in the remote desert of the Australian Outback. Besides, she had a family, responsibilities, events planned. Then she started having the dreams—dreams of an old, very black woman with tightly curled gray hair and a great round-cheeked smile. She became aware of Outback Steakhouse advertisements and posters for Australian trips everywhere. Out of the blue, one of her friends gave her a stuffed kangaroo. She was held up in traffic over and over—always behind Subaru Outbacks. When it's important, the universe can be darn persistent.

She finally got the message—*You are supposed to go to Australia!*—and agreed to come.

So here we were on a plane together. Not only were we on our way to a continent halfway around the world, but from the materials I had received in advance, I knew we were really going to be roughing it: sleeping in the open air in sleeping bags on the ground.

I had no idea what this adventure would bring. I knew from Gary that the Aborigines—although disguised as a primitive culture—were incredibly advanced in their healing practices and psychic abilities. I knew they were the oldest continuous culture on the planet. At least 60,000 years old! That's 60,000 years of continually passing on their wisdom. Imagine the wisdom you gain from your one life experience or from a few days of sitting with a wise elder in their seventies or eighties. Now imagine the knowledge to be gained from a culture that has passed that wisdom down from generation to generation, a culture intimately connected to nature. Imagine the wisdom to be gained from more than 60,000 years of living deeply connected to the Earth.

I was half excited and half terrified.

I had deliberately come with little knowledge of the people, the country, or the surroundings. I wanted my mind to be free of any Western cultural prejudices concerning the Aborigines and what I was about to experience. At the last minute I grabbed a book about Australia and was reading it on the twenty-one-hour flight.

That's when I learned that the Australian Outback has the largest and most poisonous snakes and spiders in the world.

49

LIGHT FOR
THE LIGHTWORKERS

We arrived in Australia a week before the ceremonies were scheduled. We stayed with John's friends—Quinton and Angela. They had a beautiful woodsy bungalow in the rolling hills near Brisbane. A large covered veranda ran around the house, and the whole place had a warm, homey feeling with its weathered, unfinished wood siding on the outside and wood paneling on the inside. It was all deliberately decorated to blend naturally with the terrain. Even the single-wide trailer next to the house, where Karyn and I stayed, had been given a mossy sloping roof and a porch trimmed with bamboo. Trees sheltered the trailer and house, growing close to the walls.

The surrounding woods were sparse and opened often to rolling brown hillsides—so different from the thick undergrowth and trees in the Pacific Northwest.

Because they were John's friends, of course Quinton and Angela were amazing people, deeply connected to Spirit and the Earth. Gorgeous bright birds and wild turkeys were always around the feeders that surrounded the house. Every night a new group of interesting people would drop by. We would sit on the veranda or inside the house, amid the sacred art and riotous plants, and the conversation and laughter would flow. Sometimes, I would lead meditations and Karyn would channel Divine Mother.

Quinton and Angela entertained us generously during the days. They knew I loved dolphins, so one day they took us to feed dolphins in Tin Can Bay. On the way back we stopped at Great Sandy National Park with its immense trees. They were ten feet in diameter with great buttresslike fins growing out from the bottom and vines growing up the sides like Faberge filigree. It was in this park that I encountered a wild five-foot-long iguana (pronounced "go-anna" in Australia) while having lunch. Now I have never been afraid of animals and I loved this wild creature.

I asked Quinton, "Can you feed them?" not realizing that Australians have a rather unique sense of humor.

"Sure you can," he replied, completely straight-faced, probably thinking, *You can feed them your hand.*

I held out a piece of my sandwich for the iguana. He was more than happy to take it—along with my index finger. As a matter of fact the finger was probably more attractive than the sandwich because it was fresher. No, no, he didn't bite it off. He merely closed his jaws around it. With his backward facing—and very sharp—teeth, I knew instinctively that to scream and pull would not have been the smart move.

Don't panic, I told myself. *Just wait until he's done, otherwise the two of us are gonna rip that finger right off.*

So I waited. I didn't panic. I just waited.

It hurt like hell.

I waited until he let go, and when he finally gave up, I heard his jaws actually click as they opened.

It was when he let go that it *really* hurt. But Australians are hardy, so we rinsed it in disinfectant and didn't make any more fuss.

Karyn later told me, "There's meat to that, that you were bitten by a wild iguana." *Interesting.* I have since learned that an iguana as a totem brings gifts of patience, gentleness, kindness, and understanding. Gifts

I had long been using in my healing work. Another source claimed that they are masters of contentment, confidence, contemplation, and appreciation, and that their main message is: *Don't rush. Stop being in a hurry. Everything comes in due time. Take time to simply be.* Something Gary had tried to teach me for years.

Karyn and I did a few small speaking events together while we were in Brisbane. I would lead healing meditations and Karyn would channel Divine Mother. We were a good team—I was able to get everyone relaxed and ready to hear Mother's messages. The last night we stayed with Quinton and Angela, they arranged for us to speak before a group of healers. This was a group who met every week to give their healing services to the community completely free of charge.

It was an extraordinarily spiritual group of people with wide-open hearts. They were skilled in many types of alternative medicine, various massage therapies, and energy healing.

They met in an old community center with creaky wooden floors and rough wooden walls. It had once been a theater and had a large open floor space where the seating had been, and a small stage. The healers set up a dozen or so tables, similar to massage tables. I was surprised to look out and see a long line of people at the door waiting for their help. There were people who were crippled, injured, and had all kinds of maladies. The doors opened and the healing began.

Karyn and I were going to speak at the end of the evening, so we walked around and watched for a while. Various healers reached out to us between other clients. "Would you like to hop up on the table?" We were happy to get help after our long flight and all the hiking we'd been doing.

As I moved around the room watching these healers greet and touch and help the long line of people, hour after hour, I was deeply moved by the humility and generosity of these amazing souls. I had a realization: *They have no idea how powerful they are.* They couldn't see themselves as I saw them, that they were filled with the most expansive love and compassion. It was something I needed to see, that most of us don't realize the power of our gifts.

One of the most sought-after of the group was the man who organized it. He was himself crippled, bent over with a withered leg. He only stood about four feet high. When he worked on someone, he had to jump right up on the table and then down again with both feet when he had finished. It was this man who worked with some of the strongest healing energy in the group. I could see it flowing from him. It's funny how healing energy and infirmity sometimes go together, isn't it?

When they were done, we all moved away from the massage tables and set up a couple dozen nicked and rickety wooden folding chairs in a circle in the front of the auditorium. We lowered the lights. It was Karyn's and my part of the evening. I began leading the healing meditation. It was something I had done hundreds of times before, but with this group their selfless generosity had opened a tremendous flow of light and healing energy. I was caught up in the beauty of it. When I closed the meditation, the large room was filled with an intensely beautiful healing light.

I slipped into a seat next to Karyn and tapped her gently on the knee to let her know I was finished and she could begin. This was a very special group of people, here on the other side of the globe, and I couldn't wait to see what Divine Mother would tell them.

Tonight Divine Mother had a special message: "You are lightworkers, and you are part of the great net of healing light that is woven all around the Earth. It is very important that you *feel* the interconnectedness. Like your Internet, no? The inter-net of healing light. Whether or not you are conscious of it, you are woven together. When you become aware of it, you intensify the light net around Mother Earth. It is you together who are helping Mother Earth to change. To heal. To raise the consciousness of human life on this planet. By focusing on your connections to other healers—other lightworkers—around the planet you are increasing and quickening that work."

She continued to speak for some time, then said in closing, "Thank you for the beautiful work you do, beloveds. Take good care of yourselves and know that I love you."

I love you too, I thought. Even here, halfway around the world, she was with me; she was always with me. *Thank you, Divine Mother, for helping us.*

As we were folding up the chairs and putting things away, everyone kept coming up to Karyn and me and peppering us with questions. In a strange country, in the middle of another culture, there is always the temptation to hold back—to be small—in the mistaken belief that you are being respectful. But that night, Divine Love was flowing through Karyn and me and we couldn't stay small. We let it shine. They were filled with endless questions. And Karyn and I were both surprised to discover that we had answers. We talked and talked, and I could tell from the grateful thanks and hugs that came our way that Divine Love was giving us the exact messages each person needed to hear.

Before that night, I knew that I myself had been transformed by the love and profound wisdom coming from Divine Mother and the Aborigines and through Gary and my other teachers. But I didn't suspect the depth and breadth to which the teachings had permeated me. Gradually, over the many years, the knowledge that I was loved and nurtured had seeped into my beliefs and opened my heart. I now had a deep insight into the perfection and kindness of the universe.

On this trip to the Outback those teachings spilled from both Karyn and me, as if we were brimming cups. And the gratitude and wonder with which those teachings were accepted by those around us gave me a whole new perspective on who I had become.

I had downplayed my role as a healer when working with Gary. But I couldn't hide it anymore. Sitting in that auditorium, answering questions until late into the evening, I realized I *was* a healer and a teacher. Slowly, over many years, I had become a healer and a teacher. And my soul loved it! I would soon discover that this was just the beginning.

❦

Quinton and Angela had been in charge of our schedule and done a marvelous job of ferrying us everywhere we needed to be. They had taken care of every detail. So Karyn and I didn't anticipate any problems when Quinton dropped us off at the airport the next day to catch our four-hour flight to the Uluru area. We were to meet up with the other women at a lodge there and be driven to the secret Aboriginal ceremonial grounds for our week of ceremony.

At the ticket kiosk, we couldn't get our tickets to spit out our boarding passes. An attendant noticed, came over, and fiddled for a while with our tickets and the machine. Frustrated, he looked at our tickets a little more closely. "Your flight was yesterday," he told us.

Before we could take in this disaster, he said, "No worries, ladies," and led us off to a courtesy desk to rebook our flight. As he tapped away at the computer—not at all looking like he was free of worries, in fact, looking more and more worried—I realized something.

It was no accident that we had misread our tickets. If we had read them correctly, we would never have met with that wonderful group of healers the night before. Evidently, Divine Love wanted us to meet with them very much. It was at this point in my trip that I started taking what I had to offer seriously.

The man at the ticket counter was sweating bullets trying to find us seats to the Outback. He kept at his computer keyboard for the longest time. "Well, I don't think we'll be able to get anything until tomorrow," he muttered, tapping away.

This would not work at all. We were scheduled to meet up with our group in a town near Uluru early the next morning and ride out to the ceremonial grounds. But Karyn and I were not as concerned as you might think. We both realized that we were being watched over on this trip. Spirit had important work planned for us, it seemed. We *knew* we were meant to join the Aboriginal ceremonies. So neither of us panicked.

For my part, I just watched and waited, very curious about what would happen next. I had no doubt it would all work out in a perfect way. Replacing fear with curiosity was one of the most valuable skills I had learned.

As for Karyn? Karyn has impressive spiritual gifts, one of which is that she can see and hear into other dimensions. As our ticket attendant was working, Karyn saw Archangel Michael helping the man push the computer keys. Our ticket counter attendant tapped away and paused, frowning. "Nope, there's nothing . . ."

Then (Karyn told me later), she saw Archangel Michael reach over his shoulder and press a key.

The attendant was surprised for a moment, as if the screen had not done what he expected it to, and then he said, "Oh, look at that . . . well, maybe . . ."

This happened several more times. Until finally, he breathed a sigh of relief and handed us our new boarding passes. "I found something. Your flight leaves in fifteen minutes. I'll take your luggage, and I have an attendant on the way to take you where you need to go."

I thanked him profusely, jokingly offering to name my grandchild after him if my son ever had one.

"Go right ahead," he said in his charming Australian accent. "The name's Michael."

I didn't find out until later why Karyn burst out laughing.

50

CAMPING

Uluru—that most sacred of Aboriginal ceremonial sites—is a huge sandstone monolith more than two miles long and one mile wide. It rises more than a thousand feet above the ground, but one of the most startling facts about this solid chunk of sandstone is that it extends downward into the ground for another mile and a half, out of sight.

It is difficult for people of European descent to comprehend the significance Uluru has for the Aboriginal people who live in its shadow. Uluru was formed by Ancestral Beings during the Dreamtime—a time that was the creation of everything in existence and is still creating the world and will continue to create the world so long as the universe exists. Fantastical fissures and stone forms around Uluru are said to represent the living embodiment of Ancestral Beings. To some Aborigines, Uluru is the womb of the world.

I was now flying like an arrow to participate in this week of ceremonies with Jaripuyjangu community members within sight of Uluru. The Jaripuyjangu tribe is a group of Aborigines who share a common language, social structure, and spiritual practice. Aboriginal "tribes" are not structured like Native American tribes. They do not have chiefs or medicine men. Every Aboriginal person has his or her own meaningful spiritual connection to the land with spiritual responsibilities to fulfill, responsibilities to specific Ancestral and Totemic Beings and sacred sites. Many of the Jaripuyjangu live in small settlements or communities consisting of ten to twenty-four people each, and the land around Uluru is within their territory.

It was no coincidence that it was near Uluru that Gary had stayed with members of the Jaripuyjangu in 1994. I was destined to go perform ceremony with the same tribe in the same sacred area. I would not be seeing the settlement where Gary had stayed, however. I would be with different community members of the tribe, and we would be camping at a site kept sacred for ceremony.

The Jaripuyjangu women did not live at the sacred site. They would be coming from all over to gather together and perform the women ceremonies that needed to be performed at this specific place. There would be no men involved in performing the ceremonies.

What I did not know as I flew through the air bound for this event is that there had been a serious disagreement between the men and the women of the tribe about the white women's participation.

The women of this particular tribe had gathered together and decided that it was time to share their culture by sharing their ceremonies. This was secret knowledge of the truly remote Aborigines, those who had deliberately kept themselves separate from the invading European culture. These women had known that our world was in need of healing knowledge—knowledge of how to heal each other and how to live in concert with our environment—but they had been waiting for instruction from their Dreamtime meditations. With the current problems in the world, their ways needed to be spread and taught to others. And now was the time.

The Aboriginal women decided to invite some specifically selected white women to a week of sacred ceremonies—white women who had demonstrated their commitment to learning ancient Aboriginal wisdom for the purpose of helping other people and the planet.

The Aboriginal men had strongly resisted this idea.

The white man had proved untrustworthy over countless generations: stealing their land, taking their children from them, and abolishing their language and culture. At the same time the whites were always wanting to know their ancient secrets. The Aborigines had spent centuries fiercely protecting their ancient ceremonial practices—a part of their culture that they resolved would not be taken away.

On top of that, these rites were very powerful. It wasn't only that the secrets to their ceremonies could be stolen or wouldn't be fully respected, but that when you are working with this kind of powerful energy, someone can get hurt. These ceremonies connected the people to their land and their ancestral caretakers and totems. If those relationships were damaged, the people would suffer.

But the Aboriginal women held steadfast and insisted that the time to share their knowledge was now. Their most knowledgeable elders—the ones who could most powerfully communicate to the whites—were dying. One of their most revered spiritual practitioners, Auntie Ella, might not survive another year, and many of the other elders might follow close behind her.

There were many disagreements and discussions. Finally, with great reluctance, the men decided to allow white women to participate in this one set of ceremonies and they would see. But if something inappropriate happened, there would be repercussions, possible serious harm to the tribal members who were involved. Were the women willing to risk this?

A brave Jaripuyjangu woman in the tribe named Melody, a middle-aged woman who knew the English language, stepped up. She agreed to be the go-between. She and she alone would act as the liaison between the Aboriginal women and the white women. She would take full responsibility for whatever happened. If something inappropriate happened, she was willing to place her life on the line for the consequences. That was not a metaphor—it was literal. Of course, no harm would be done to her by any member of the tribe. This was the depth of their belief in their spiritual obligations: that she could die as a consequence of an outsider breaking their ceremonial law.

I didn't know about this controversy when I accepted the invitation to the Outback. I learned of the dispute only later from Lucy, another woman headed to the gathering. Lucy, a pretty brunette decked out in true Outback gear, just happened to be sitting directly behind us on the flight from Brisbane to Uluru—the flight we were assigned after missing our flight the day before. She sat behind us again on the bus ride to the lodge where we were staying. While standing in line to check into the hotel, there she was again directly in front of us. Clearly the universe had wanted us to meet.

She approached us and asked if we were heading to the Outback ceremonies with the Aborigines. She was a native-born Australian and she instantly became a wonderful friend and helpmate.

She took us into the hotel store and helped us buy special equipment she knew we would need for camping in the Outback, including a canteen and a marvelous broad-brimmed hat with a face net that was essential in the flying-insect-infested desert to which we were headed.

Lucy was dating an Aboriginal man and joining the ceremonies to better understand his world. In hushed whispers over dinner, she filled us in on the tribal dispute. She tried to give us some inkling of the protocols we needed to follow. Because we were not part of the Jaripuyjangu tribe, we had no relationship to the members, no place in their society. So during this time, we would need to respect their autonomy and follow strict protocols in dealing with them.

The hotel was a sprawling complex of bungalows with a campground and open-air grills for the patrons to use. Lucy grilled us kangaroo, emu, and crocodile that night to "help our bodies connect to the land." Crocodile isn't bad—it tastes like steak. But let me warn you, emu is not for everybody.

I was up at dawn and saw the sunrise hit Uluru. It was freezing cold and very dark before the sun rose. In this strange flat land I was able to see Uluru's dark hulking shape clearly against the horizon. Gradually, the clouds were lit pink and purple from underneath and then—Boom!—

the sun was up and everything was bright with the clear desert light: the red earth, the sparse dottings of olive-gray trees no higher than a tall man, the parched yellow tufts of grass, and the rustling white skeletons of dried flowers. Behind the undulating land, Uluru loomed red-orange against the white sky, an impossibly massive presence.

Within a few hours we were loading our gear into Jeeps and 4x4s for the trek to the Aboriginal ceremonial grounds.

John had put me in contact with Emerald and Gina, two white Australian women who had established a long-term relationship with the women of the Jaripuyjangu. They had made many arrangements for the rest of us who were coming from far away. They supplied the heavier equipment like sleeping bags and the canvas covers for the bags, a kitchen camper, a portable water tower, basic food—many things to make this collaboration possible. They were wonderful, dedicated women.

As we drove over rough road, Emerald coached us in the protocols for our time with the Aborigines. These restrictions may sound severe, but the Aborigines believe that their laws governing the correct way to conduct ceremony have been laid down by Ancestral Beings since the Dreamtime. Many of their stories are moral tales about what happens to individuals who break ceremonial protocols. This was a powerful ceremonial site and we were trespassers on the land of these Ancestral Beings.

Absolutely no photographs were allowed.

No electronic devices at all were to be used.

The Aboriginal women had already established their campground and the ceremonial grounds. Our camp would be nearby, but completely separate.

We were not to approach their camp unless invited.

We were not to approach the Aboriginal women or try to talk with them or give them gifts directly.

We were not even to meet their eyes unless they initiated the contact.

During ceremony, if we were not dancing, we were to place our-selves on the ground at a level beneath any Aboriginal woman who was performing in the ceremony.

By participating in these sacred rites, we were taking a vow never to reveal the details of the dances, songs, paintings, and sacred gestures that were part of the ceremonies.

Did we all agree? We did.

I fervently hoped I could remember all these protocols.

We bounced along through a terrain that left me feeling like I had landed on Mars. We were surrounded by red desert sand and sparse dry vegetation for miles, no sign of civilization save for the rutted, bumpy dirt road. After about forty-five minutes, we came to a wire fence and a gate with a sign saying "Do not cross. Protected Aboriginal Land." We passed through the gate and drove on from there to the camp.

The Aboriginal women's camp was already established. Out of the corner of my eye, I noticed that it was not so very different from a gath-ering of American campers. The tents were brightly colored and syn-thetic. There were some campfire pits prepared for cooking and logs placed around on which to sit.

We were told to set up our sleeping bags wherever we liked on the other side of Melody's tent, away from the Aborigines' side. It was as if our camps were separated by an invisible line with Melody's tent in the middle. She was our "middle man," in a physical as well as figurative sense.

As we went about setting up our side of the camp, I was becoming nervous, frightened even. It was a harsh, strange red land. I could hear the tribe's odd-sounding language float across the divide every so often. Although the Jeep ride from the hotel to this remote camp on restricted grounds was only about an hour, civilization felt very far away—like I had stepped in to a place outside of time. I could not have been more isolated, more outside everything with which I was comfortable and familiar. The dire warnings we had received during the protocol coaching had struck home. I had no idea what was going to happen during these ceremonies.

Maybe I should have thought this through more thoroughly.

Back in June, it had seemed like a great idea to join the Aborigines in ceremony. Now that I was finally here, months later, it was really frightening.

There was no "campground" per se. Separate areas had been selected for the Aboriginal and non-Aboriginal participants, but on both sides our sleeping bags and tents were in desert not much different looking from all the surrounding desert: a few sparse trees, dry tufts of grass, the red bare earth.

The ceremonial area—the dance grounds—was located on the Aboriginal side of the imaginary line separating the two camping areas. It was a natural clearing in which they had placed five enormous bonfire pits.

The kitchen Emerald and Gina had provided for both camps was set up off to the side next to a small water tower. We white women set up two fire pits on our side with logs around them on which to sit. This is where we non-Aboriginals would gather during the days, to talk and share food, when no ceremonies were taking place.

We never saw or heard any actual men. Even though I had been told they were near, I never saw the slightest sign of them. They set up a camp somewhere in a location that was never disclosed, at least to us. The men's job was to contain the spiritual energy to keep us grounded and safe. We had been told the ceremonial dances were potentially dangerous. I had no idea what that meant, and it increased my apprehension.

Ranging in age from their early twenties to middle sixties, most of the white women were from Australia. Karyn and I were the only women from the United States. There was a young woman in her early twenties from Canada who appeared to have traveled extensively, and another woman from Canada named Sue who was a teacher. As we set up camp everyone seemed to be happy and excited. They didn't seem to be apprehensive despite the harsh environment, and despite not knowing what lay ahead. I came to know them all as amazingly coura-geous women.

A few of the Aboriginal women came out to watch us establishing our campsites. I spotted some ladies near the water tank and noticed that they talked excitedly to each other and seemed to be indicating Karyn. I found out later that they were saying, "That's her. That's the one we've been talking to in the Dreamtime."

Right away I noticed that the red earth of this land stained every-thing it touched. Years later, my nightgown and socks were still stained after many washings. Yes, I brought a nightgown to the desert. That's how much of a bushwhacker I was.

Karyn and I chose to set up our little campsite on the very outskirts of the white women's area. While I set up equipment, I asked Karyn to please do something about the swarms of ants. They were huge and there were millions of them crawling all over the land. Their enormous ant hills were visible everywhere—dirt piled more than five feet high—with ants constantly crawling over the surface of each hill.

Karyn did a ceremony the minute we chose our campsite, setting out an offering of honey for the ants at one of the hills. She somehow made an agreement with them that we would respect them if they would respect the small space we were taking up for only a few days. As it turned out, Karyn and I were the only white women that did not have problems with ants in our campsite.

I put up the tent where Karyn and I would change clothes and keep our supplies. Then I put our sleeping bags into "swags." The swags were heavy canvas bags into which the sleeping bags were inserted. At night we would get into our sleeping bag within the swag, pull the flap of the swag over our face and head, and—voila—instant one-person tent. Sort of. It was what everyone had been supplied with, but I couldn't help thinking that there would be nothing to keep out the poisonous snakes and spiders should they choose to crawl in with me.

Maybe I should have thought this through more thoroughly.

51

SACRED FIRES

I felt completely surrounded by fire and movement. It was my first night in the desert Outback, and I was sitting on the ground, clothed only in a long black skirt and walking shoes, my body painted as living canvas—my own skin transformed into a spiritual connection to the Dreamtime.

I could see shining black faces, blond hair, arms and large breasts painted with swirls and dots—the whole scene lit by five massive bonfires. The Aboriginal women were dancing with mesmerizing movements. Outside the cavorting firelight it was pitch-black night.

The fires leaped and crackled.

Wooden clappers beat out complex rhythms as the Aboriginal women performed their secret and sacred ceremony.

The pale faces belonging to us white women seemed to glow with an alien shine in the firelight as if the light of the sacred fires was saying, *Look who is here. Who are these strangers from across mountains and seas?*

We were indeed here, and we were expected to participate, not just watch. Spectators were strictly forbidden. Yet I didn't know what was expected of me. There was deep spiritual work being done here in this harshest of lands—life and death were hanging in the balance. Our liaisons had impressed that upon us.

For several reasons, it was hard to make out who was present and what was around. First, the desert darkness was solid and everything was lit by competing firelight and shadow. Even though the enormous bonfires were about five feet in diameter, I could only see a few feet by their light. I knew there were twenty white women and about twenty-three to twenty-five Aboriginal women in the ceremony, but not everyone was visible to me. At times I had the feeling that there were many more people than that present.

The second reason I couldn't tell what was going on was my fear of breaking protocols. We were not to look the Aborigines directly in the eye while they were performing ceremony. That was a sign of disrespect. They were allowed to look you in the eye first, but if they did not deliberately catch your eye, you were to avoid direct eye contact.

Not wanting to offend them, I barely looked up, afraid to break the protocol. But I gathered plenty of images by looking out of my peripheral vision. And of course I could hear. There was singing in a language stranger than any I had ever heard. The only accompanying instruments were special sticks with ash-burned markings clacked against each other. Then there was the dancing—repetitive and hypnotic.

We had all been coached that when Melody called out "Ceremony!" we were to spring into action. This was the call to join the Aborigines at the dance grounds. We white women were to throw on long black skirts and nothing else, no top—only protective shoes and an optional hat. We needed to respond immediately. To dawdle would be considered the height of disrespect.

We were to be ready at any time because there was no predicting when ceremony would happen, whether it was noon or darkness. Ceremony would happen when the Aboriginal elders sensed that the conditions were right. This was a tribe that lived in the present moment, not on any schedule. The natural rhythms of the Earth and Ancestral Beings dictated when it was time for ceremony, not our desires.

The generalities that I am disclosing here are not a violation of my commitment to keep the ceremonies secret. It is the details of the painting, the songs, and the dances that I am forbidden to share.

During my stay at this sacred site the Jaripuyjangu women did not teach us spirituality through lecture. The community did not speak English to me. In fact, I rarely even saw an adult Jaripuyjangu woman outside of ceremony. They stayed on their side of the ceremonial grounds and we stayed on ours. We met in the middle to participate in ceremony together. Everything I learned was experiential. Therefore, my reporting here is not intended to be an anthropological study. It is an account of my own experiences and what I took away.

During this ceremony, which took place on our first night, I was surprised and also relieved to see a dog roaming on the sidelines of the dancing. This one was a scrawny midsize dog, a dingo as it turned out. He did not seem alarmed by the presence of the white strangers. Somehow seeing him brought me comfort. Evidently, a love of animals transcended cultural differences.

The ceremony finished and we went back to our camp. As I left the dance grounds, I saw a few young children running around in the Aboriginal women's camp. Of course there would be children, I thought. These are real women from a real tribe living their real lives, not some tourist show. At the introduction of these elements we humans all share—a love of children, companion animals—I began to relax.

Our camp fell quickly asleep after the long day, but I woke in the middle of the night having to go to the bathroom. There I lay with nothing but a bag-within-a-bag between me and the inhospitable desert—poisonous snakes, spiders as big as platters, wild camels, feral pigs, and freezing cold. It took me an hour and a half to work up the nerve to leave the bag. Then I walked into the pitch black, dug a trench, relieved my full bladder, filled in the hole, bagged my used toilet paper, and scurried back to my sleeping bag, shivering with cold and clutching my TP.

Maybe I should have thought this through more thoroughly.

After the initial ceremony around the bonfires the first night, there wasn't another call to ceremony for a long time.

Day after day, we white women waited, battling the heat during the day, the cold at night, and the insects that came in waves, a different species for every time of day. I had to be very careful not to touch any of the fallen wood with my bare hands. Firewood and even the logs we had gathered to sit on around the campfire were baked so hard by the desert heat that they would fill my hands with splinters at the merest brush.

The hat with a net that tied over my face, the one that Lucy had instructed me to buy back at the lodge, was indispensable. The insects were so thick in the air at times that they would get in your eyes, your nostrils, and your mouth. My hat protected my face. Another indispensable item was Chapstick. I can't imagine what my lips would have become without it. It was so dry, I seemed to use a tube a day. It wasn't water I ran out of—it was Chapstick. I had to ration it toward the end.

There were no showers. In that heat you can imagine how our appearance altered as the days went by. Our hair became impossibly dirty and matted. Our bodies continually smeared with the fine red dirt. Actually, there was a marvelous sense of freedom in not wearing makeup and in not caring about how dirty my hair or my clothes were. Here in the desert with deep spiritual work being done, appearance was irrelevant, and I was surprised how good that felt.

I had steeled myself to eat honey ants, grubs, and bugs, as Gary had, but in the end I survived mostly on cheese sandwiches, which were part of the food brought in by Emerald and Gina to stock the kitchen.

Gradually I became aware that, during this downtime, the Aborigines were preparing us for what was to come.

I could feel energetic and subconscious changes and I could see them in my companions as well. They were opening us energetically, removing blockages and repairing our mental, emotional, physical, and etheric bodies. They were working on us in the Dreamtime at the energetic-patterning level.

Many of the white women were breaking down and releasing long-held pain and worry during the slow, hot days. And for some reason, many of them sought out Karyn or me to talk with during this processing. There would often be two little clutches of women, one gathered around Karyn at one end of our camp and one gathered around me at the other. Karyn and I were really surprised to find ourselves teaching the teachers and helping to heal the healers. We didn't know how much knowledge we held until we were put in this group of amazing, knowledgeable women and they kept seeking us out for counsel. It was really an eye-opener for both Karyn and me, a taste of what was to come as we started to bring everything we had learned out into the world.

One of the important things I learned on that trip is that no matter how extraordinary a life a woman is living, no matter how much we are accomplishing, most of us feel inadequate.

This was brought home to me while talking one day with a woman named Heather, a slim blonde who was stunningly attractive even while sporting her matted, dirty hair. We sat together warming ourselves at the fire one chilly morning in our camping area.

Heather was a remarkable woman. She was a marathon runner in her midforties. With her husband, she ran an alternative energy company that was supplying impoverished women around the world with solar-powered cooking stoves. She told me she had three small children under the age of ten.

After I had extracted all this information, Heather confided in me, "I don't know what's wrong with me." She sounded truly perplexed. "I don't know why I'm so tired all the time. I feel like I'm letting my husband down by not being able to do more."

She was a mother, an athlete, and a businesswoman. She was doing all these astounding things, but she didn't see why she might be tired! She just kept demanding more of herself.

Why? Why are we so unappreciative and judgmental of ourselves? If there is any message I received over and over from Gary, from Divine Mother, from my celestial team, it was this: *Embrace and love and accept yourself just as you are. Accept all of you, especially the parts you dislike. When you embrace every part of yourself, even the unwanted parts—only then can you truly shine.*

At the same time I shared these ideas with Heather, my inner wisdom was teaching them to me. As always, the best way to learn something is to teach it.

One night, I awoke suddenly in the early hours. Behind my closed eyes, I saw patterns of Aboriginal symbols. It was like when you stare at something and then close your eyes. What you see behind your lids is the negative of what you were looking at—the white areas are black, and black areas are white. The images I saw were like that, a snapshot negative that quickly faded away to be replaced by another. Although I didn't recognize the shapes, they reminded me of the Aboriginal paintings I had seen: elaborate stories told with dots and squiggles.

I instinctively knew that this was a sign that the Aborigines were working on me—I was being healed by the Aborigines. They were sending transmissions, upgrading my software, so to speak, and removing what didn't serve me anymore. They were raising my energetic vibration for the ceremonies we would be performing together that week. I knew the tribe was helping me to grow in consciousness. My willingness to be there and experience their wisdom had given them permission to help me. I was grateful for it although I didn't yet understand all that their work entailed or how long it would go on. For many years, I would occasionally wake up in the middle of the night and see remnants of Aboriginal patterns and squiggles in my mind's eye before they quickly faded away.

At the same time, Karyn was also taking care of her own spiritual health. One night she was feeling particularly spacey. She had been absorbing so much, things seemed to be spinning around for her. She wanted to ground and integrate.

Most of the other women, including me, had gone to bed. With the intention of creating a sacred fire, she threw some tobacco into our campfire and began to pray for counsel. She asked for guidance and help in understanding everything that was going on here in the Outback.

Suddenly, an enormous furry tarantula crawled out of the desert into the light of her fire. It was the size of a dinner plate, fully eight inches across with a body the size of her fist. It was probably what is known as a "barking spider" to the locals.

She uttered a not-very-sacred expletive.

Thinking it didn't know she was there, she flicked some dirt at it with her foot. This caused the tarantula to leap high into the air directly toward her. Jumping to her feet, she ran. The spider pursued.

It chased her several times around the campfire until she gained a little ground and had the fire between herself and it. She dodged to one side; the tarantula moved to cut her off. She dodged to the other side; it countered.

It was at this point that it occurred to her that this was not normal behavior, even in Australia. Although the creature was large for a spider, it was still a hundred times smaller than herself. She put her hands on her hips and said aloud, "What do you want from me?"

The tarantula replied, in her mind, *What do you want from ME? You're the one who called me here.*

Ahhhhh. Counsel. You just never know how things are going to show up in the Outback. "Thank you for coming to help me. What do you have to teach me?" she asked.

After they had telepathically conferred, the spider returned to its burrow, probably grumbling about being disturbed in the middle of the night.

Thankfully, I slept through the whole thing.

After that waiting period, the ceremonies resumed and continued to build during the remaining days. When Melody called "Ceremony!" we all came running to the Aborigines' side of the camp.

I found myself breaking protocols left and right. Most of the time, I didn't even know it was a protocol until I broke it.

For example, at one of the first ceremonies the Aborigines were teaching us the dance. The movement was so strange to me, I just couldn't get the hang of it. That was not a problem. The Aboriginal women were very understanding and patient. But out of embarrassment, I started to laugh out loud at myself. A young Aboriginal woman, who was watching from beside the fire, quickly gave me a look that said: *No laughing.* It was not appropriate to laugh while in ceremony or even in preparation for it.

In spite of our ignorance, we outsiders gradually became active participants in the ceremonies. There was some brief teaching (as with the dance steps above), but for the most part we learned by doing, by being drawn up by the participating women and encouraged to join in. This was not a weekend workshop—it was work-study all the way. Energetic healing was being done for the participants, the tribe, and the Earth. Connections were being made to the natural environment, connections that would provide the food and water that would sustain the tribe through the coming summer. In this harsh, unforgiving land, life and death were literally in the balance. We were expected to contribute as we could. Where the ceremony called for it, the Aboriginal women painted us just as they painted themselves, using our bodies as the canvas. We sometimes contributed to the rhythms, the dancing, and the energetic enlivening.

The energies that we tapped into together had great power. There was no room for mistakes even out of ignorance.

One of our group was taking pictures of our side of the camp. She took out her cell phone and took a picture of the kitchen area that separated the two camps. Melody came running up, extremely upset. She yelled at the woman, telling her that she didn't understand the serious consequences involved—that Melody's very life could be in jeopardy. The white woman was understandably shaken because she didn't realize she was violating the rules. There were no people in the picture. It was only a photo of the kitchen. But evidently the land itself—the surrounding desert, the very ground—was sacred and not to be photographed.

It made me realize how serious this gathering was and that Melody was indeed terrified of the consequences of any misbehavior on our parts.

52

A MOTHER'S LOVE

"Ceremony!"

I was restfully napping, when I was startled into consciousness by a loud call.

"Ceremony!" It came again.

With my eyes still closed and my mind in an overheated fog, I tried to decipher the sounds I was hearing. *What's going on?* I slowly opened my eyes, and the orange tarp I saw directly above me was completely unfamiliar. *Where the heck am I?*

I heard frantic voices yelling things I couldn't quite make out. Stretching my eyes wide open, as if that would bring me awake, I heard a pan drop off in the distance. People were running past in a mad dash, their shoes muffled by the soft sand. *I remember now. I'm in the Outback.* I had taken refuge for a nap in the middle of the day in our supply tent.

My hazy thoughts were interrupted by the sound of the metal zipper of the tent being quickly unzipped. The orange tent flap was thrown open and the glaring sun shone directly into my eyes. "Ugh!" I said.

Karyn's head, her black hair matted with dust, poked through the opening. Still breathless from running, she panted, "Hurry up. They're calling 'Ceremony!'"

Ceremony! I yanked off my cotton short-sleeve shirt, formerly beige and now stained red. Naked except for my floor-length black polyester skirt, I grabbed my shoes, also stained with red dust. Once outside the tent I wrestled with the zipper. I was tempted to just forget it, but we needed to keep the ants and other desert critters out of our food.

As I raced to the ceremony grounds, I saw I was racing alone. Everyone else had already arrived.

I immediately plopped to the soft sand on the outside of the circle of white women earnestly watching a half-dozen Aboriginal women dancing and singing in an indecipherable chant.

Everyone was clapping along to the beat of the singing, the white women with their hands and a few of the Aborigines with their wooden clapping sticks. I folded my legs underneath me and started clapping, caught up in the simple but captivating rhythms.

It was one of our final days with the Aborigines. Even though the meaning of each ceremony remained a mystery to me, I was able to sense that the ceremonies were mounting in significance and power.

I watched as the Aborigines danced in bare feet on the burning hot sand. A kind of awe began building inside me. I closed my eyes and gently rocked to the hypnotic cadence. It felt like my worries and concerns were being slowly melted away by the rhythm of the clappers. With my eyes still closed, the music seemed to fade quietly into the background and I focused on my heart. I could feel gratitude welling up inside me . . . deep gratitude for my life . . . all of it, even the painful parts.

The gratitude in my heart seemed to grow and grow until its warmth engulfed my entire body. I found myself caught up in a wave of overwhelming love and gratitude to Gaia. In that moment, I could feel a deep love from Mother Earth extending to all of her creation. Rocking to the gentle rhythm of the Aboriginal song, I understood that we were Gaia's children whom she lovingly provides for, nurtures, and shelters. Feeling the depth of her unending selfless love brought tears to my eyes.

I felt like I was a young child finally waking up to the intense love a doting parent held for me. Gaia had always been abundantly providing for my needs. Despite my lack of respect, acknowledgment, and even occasional abuse, Gaia's love for me had never wavered. I was one of her children, a beloved part of her. The realization of the utter depth of Gaia's undying love almost took my breath away. I became aware that tears were streaming down my face as I felt Mother Earth's love penetrate my every cell.

I bathed in that radiant nurturing love for a long time, eventually opening my eyes. One of the Aboriginal elders was looking directly at me, her eyes shining. With a grateful smile I nodded to her, and she continued to meet my eyes, smiling broadly.

I realized that she saw it. She knew that their ceremony had helped me recognize what they had always known . . . a mother's deep love for me and for all of her children.

53

THUNDERSTORMS

It wasn't all waiting and ceremony. Some of the sweetest moments of my time there involved the Aboriginal children.

The Aboriginal women seldom ventured outside their camp and the ceremonial grounds—with three exceptions: our liaison Melody and two Aboriginal girls who appeared to be free to roam wherever they liked. The young girls both knew a little bit of English. They could be seen sometimes in the outdoor kitchen area or by the large elevated water tank at the edge of the two camps.

There was a tall Aboriginal girl named Judith who looked to be about thirteen or fourteen. She was always smiling, shyly sitting in the background. The other girl was much younger, a dark-skinned girl with blond hair who appeared to be around four or five years old. Her name was Margaret—a sweet, sweet girl.

I often volunteered to carry the heavy containers of water for the kitchen in the hopes I would meet an Aborigine at the water tank. Judith, the older girl, often hung around there. I watched her out of the corner of my eye and I'm sure she was doing the same with me. We both looked and sounded so foreign to each other. As time went by, she became bolder and would walk beside me as I went about my water carrying.

Little Margaret seemed to be comfortable in either camp and would also sometimes accompany me, grinning and curious. More than once, she reached out and affectionately rubbed my arm, a look of wonder on her face. Out of respect for the Aborigines, I didn't speak to the children or seek them out unless they came to me first. But what a joy when they walked up to me and wanted my company.

Because of the heat of the desert, I was always drinking water. I carried a big green water canteen I had bought back at the lodge (ironically, it had "Made in the US" stamped on the bottom). One day the youngest one, Margaret, walked along beside me. She was curious about the water canteen that I had strapped over my shoulder. I took the canteen off and squirted the water from it into her mouth. She gleefully exclaimed, "Rainwater!"

I let her carry the canteen around with her for several hours after that, but eventually I had to ask her for it back. She dutifully handed it over. Even though I could not take her picture, I have a picture of an Aboriginal child who looks like Margaret's twin on my altar. I often look at it and think, "Rainwater!"

The ceremonies built in intensity toward the end of our time together, each one more powerful than the one before it.

After the previous day's ceremony, I was still walking around in a glow of gratitude to Mother Earth. Today was our last day for ceremony. I tried not to have expectations, but I sensed something big was about to happen. I spent most of the morning wondering what it would be.

"Ceremony! Ceremony!" Melody yelled from the far end of the camp.

Looks like I'm about to find out, I thought, as I pulled off my clothes and stepped into my dusty black skirt. Determined not to be late for ceremony today, still yanking up my skirt I ran toward the Aborigines' side of the camp.

Uncharacteristically, I was one of the first to arrive at the ceremony site this time. Women were just starting to assemble. I sat front and center at the edge of the ceremony site where the Aborigines would be dancing in front of us. *Best seat in the house,* I thought. *How perfect for my last day.*

It didn't take long for the other women to arrive. We were all naked except for our long black skirts. Gazing around, I marveled at seeing such a wide range of radiant skin colors represented. Between the white women and the Aboriginal women, we were fair skinned to dark ebony and everything in between.

I shifted my legs underneath me as I settled my body into the sandy dirt. The Aborigines started singing again in their native tongue. A few of the white participants started clapping to the sound of the beat. It was fascinating watching the Aboriginal dancers. Despite the discomfort of sitting in the hot sun with my back aching, I was spellbound. I couldn't understand what the Aborigines were singing, but through their powerful song and dance they were able to convey gratitude again. From where I sat a few yards away from the dancing, I felt the warmth intensifying inside me as it had the day before. Huge waves of gratitude were welling up and rippling through my body.

I noticed a large dragonfly hovering close to the head of one of the dancing Aborigines. As I stared at it, the dragonfly seemed to blend into the leaves of the scraggly trees behind it, as if it were part of the landscape. Then I noticed that the same thing was happening with the dancing Aborigines. They were blending into the background of large red rocks and puffy white clouds in the bright blue sky.

Everything shimmered and seemed to melt together. Although I could distinctly see each object, it felt as if there was no separation between them. With everything blended together as one, I couldn't feel any demarcations or distinguish any lines. Each person and object blended or rolled off infinitely into the next and the next and the next. I felt a sense of boundless interconnectedness between everything.

What happened next was even more profound. My heart began to expand until it expanded far beyond my body. I felt intense love and compassion flowing from it. An airy feeling came over me, as if there were no time and space. This went beyond any intellectual knowing there was no time and space—I could *feel* there was no time and space! I lost all sense of where I began and ended. And all sense of time passing. It felt like everything was interconnected in a timeless, boundless consciousness. And I knew, with the kind of knowing that encompasses your whole being, that I was part of this infinite consciousness. In an instant I knew this One-Consciousness wasn't only within me and everything around me, it stretched infinitely beyond the cosmos, beyond our universe. The intensity of the love coming from this interconnected consciousness struck me to the heart.

After several minutes, I took a deep breath and placed my hands on my heart. *Thank you, thank you, thank you, my dear Aboriginal brethren, for helping me to feel the loving consciousness that is a part of me,* I silently said.

Pulling my knees up toward my chest, I wrapped my arms around my legs and basked in the delicious glow of the moment. I leaned my cheek against my knees, closed my eyes, and listened to the beautiful singing with indiscernible lyrics but a meaning I could clearly feel in my heart.

As the ceremony wound to a close, we walked back in silence to our campground. A half-hour later I headed over to the open-air kitchen to see if I could help out with anything. As I approached the makeshift kitchen—three long tables and a portable cookstove—a loud *ping* caught my attention. There was a second loud *ping* as another heavy raindrop hit the metal roof of the chuck wagon that held our food supplies. Within seconds, the metal roof was filled with loud dancing raindrops bouncing off the top. As a loud crack of thunder sounded overhead, I ran to take shelter in the supply tent I shared with Karyn. I was caught in a downpour before I reached the tent. The warm rain felt so good against my dirty hair and skin, I reached out my arms, closed my eyes, and looked up at the dark clouds overhead and let it pour over me.

The storms were intense and lasted for many hours.

We watched the thunderstorms for a long time, through the afternoon and evening. It was a tremendous downpour. We watched the rolling purple, blue, and gray clouds and sheets of rain circling the camp. It poured on us for a while and then moved off across the flat desert to the horizon, the lightning flashes and rumbles reaching us from far away. Then the storm turned and approached the camp again. As it hit, we ducked for cover and crowded inside the truck and Jeep like clowns stuffed in a circus car.

This pattern repeated over and over. Sometimes we stood outside and enjoyed the rain on our matted hair and filthy bodies. I rinsed my hair in the rain from the downpour off the tarp on the truck. It took off the first layer or two, anyway.

The children loved playing in the mud and running in the rain. When the clouds moved away, we stood on top of the truck to see Uluru in its glorious purple color. In this land of constant sun, Uluru was normally colored orange. Seeing it in its purple regalia was a rare sight.

The rain went on into the night. I remember a few of us diehards standing in the rain at night by the ceremonial campfire that still burned on, sputtering and spitting. Such fun and excitement. For the Aborigines there is also a spiritual aspect to thunderstorms. The lightning is to rebalance the world and the rain is to cleanse. I think all of us felt the renewal.

I learned later, from a hotel clerk, that the desert had not seen such storms for many years. Karyn told me that the Aboriginal women felt the white women's spiritual energy had greatly improved the strength of this year's storms.

54

A BLESSING

By now you are getting the idea that Karyn is a very special woman. It's true. Because she was telepathic, she had been connecting to the elders of this Aboriginal group for weeks before we got there. That's why they had been smiling, nodding, and pointing at her that first day, as if to say, "That's her."

On the last day of our stay, Karyn came to find me, all excited. We had been given the privilege of visiting the revered Aboriginal elder, Auntie Ella, in her tent! It was something few white women had done or were going to do.

To appreciate this honor, you have to realize that we neophytes among the white women had only seen the adult Aboriginal women during ceremony. A few in our camp had had the honor of bringing them meals and some had presented gifts of clothing and fun "girl stuff" to some of the tribe members they saw out and about, but other than that there hadn't been much social contact. We had been lectured very severely about that on the way out here. The Aboriginal women needed to minimize their interactions with us, especially during this time of ceremony, because it was a time of intense focus for them.

There were three different communities of Jaripuyjangu women represented here. We had been blessed to have several powerful medicine women present, and Auntie Ella was the most revered. Now Karyn and I were getting a private audience. I was excited . . . and terrified.

For Karyn, however, it was different. She had been communicating with them in the Dreamtime. And because they knew her, she was allowed to sometimes go with Emerald to visit on the Aboriginal side of camp.

Before we left the states, Karyn and I had arranged for our spiritual communities to prepare gifts. The community members worked to prepare the gifts with the specific intention of sending love to the Aboriginal community in Australia. We gathered and strung bead necklaces. We bought Native American blankets—as many as we could manage to carry with us in our limited luggage. In addition, Angela and Quinton had taken us to collect beautiful white feathers, which the Aborigines prized highly for use in ceremony. Everything had been blessed and prepared with love.

Auntie Ella knew all this and wanted to accept our gifts with special thanks.

So, in the middle of the afternoon I found myself on the Aboriginal side of the camp, bearing gifts. We reached Auntie Ella's small four-person tent and crawled in. I didn't know what the protocols were, so I stayed on my knees, immediately sat down as soon as I was inside the tent, and kept my gaze downward.

There wasn't much in the tent: a few unidentifiable belongings, sleeping bags, and blankets stacked around. Auntie Ella was there with a big grin on her face, sitting on the floor. She was talking in their strange language and gesturing in a broad friendly way.

I was surprised to see Judith, the teenage Aboriginal girl I had befriended, sitting beside Auntie Ella. Here, in this tent beside Auntie, she had a totally different demeanor—more responsible. Karyn explained to me that this humble and shy girl was the elder's granddaughter and destined to be a spiritual leader. I had had no idea. It was like finding out the boy you befriended at the stables was a crown prince. I realized what an honor it had been to have her take an interest in me.

We presented our gifts and Auntie Ella looked around for gifts to give us. The Aborigines are very generous and will give you whatever they have, even if they are using it or need it. I sensed she was giving us her everyday possessions, of which she had very few. She selected a small tin can of medicine and gave it to me. Then she gave me two of the wooden clappers I had seen used in the ceremonial dancing. But most surprising of all was her next gift. She handed me a small wooden iguana statue with burned markings. I looked into her face and met her eyes, they held an almost mischievous humor. Evidently, Auntie Ella agreed with Karyn. My encounter with iguana when he had nearly taken off my finger had special meaning.

After Karyn received her gifts, Auntie Ella extended her arms to me, indicating it was okay to give her a hug. As she put her arms around me, I suddenly burst into tears. I don't know where it came from but I was completely overcome by a huge, unexpected wave of gratitude. I heard myself saying, "Thank you for healing my husband, thank you for healing my husband, I am so very grateful."

Auntie Ella, a big woman, held me to her large breasts and rocked me like a loving mother. There was such a tenderness about her, and a joy. I was enveloped.

I found myself choking out, "My husband, he wanted to teach your healing ways. He wrote a book. He's been speaking and teaching workshops. And now he's dead. Shall I carry on? Do you want me to go forward?" I don't know why I was asking this. I knew she didn't speak English.

Then Auntie Ella pulled back and looked directly into my eyes. In a heavily accented patois she said, "You have our blessing."

They were passing the torch to me. They were enlisting me as they had enlisted Gary.

It was only after receiving this wonderful blessing and placing it firmly in my heart that I realized:

Auntie Ella had been able to speak English all along!

55

REBIRTH FROM
THE WOMB OF ULURU

Our time in the Outback was finished. The Aboriginal women had already packed and left, presumably joining the men in their secret location and returning to their various homes.

As we were cleaning the grounds to make sure we left no sign of our stay, I noticed a large pile of clothing and other items the Aborigines had left behind. It included many of the gifts the other women had given them. I was a bit taken aback at the waste of leaving this tall pile of perfectly good, still usable items. Then I realized that they couldn't possibly carry these things with them. They had a lifestyle of simplicity, without an emphasis on material wealth. They lived in the moment. Letting go of "baggage" that isn't serving you is part of that. They enjoyed it, then left it behind, knowing we invited participants would clear it all away from the sacred grounds as we had promised to do.

Minutes before the first group of us were to board the covered truck back to the hotel, I found myself compelled to go for a walk in the brush by myself.

This land no longer felt strange. I couldn't imagine why I had been frightened when I first arrived. It had been such an honor to be invited to this time with the Aborigines. The beautiful bodies dancing in the firelight came to mind and I knew I would be seeing those images for the rest of my life.

Suddenly, the picture of the poster of Australia that had hung in Gary's exercise room came to my mind. And in that moment, I knew. I knew that this trip had been Gary's special gift to me. Clear and strong the message hit me. *This is Gary's way of saying good-bye. Our time together as a romantic couple is ending. It's time to stop grieving and considering myself a married woman.* How dramatic and loving of him.

He knew—of course, he knew—about John Mendel. Gary knew that someone had had a romantic interest in me and I had rejected it out of hand, that I wasn't open to another romantic love. Suddenly, here in this barren desert, physically emptied but spiritually tuned up, I knew Gary was saying, *Go. Move on with your life, my dear. It's okay to love again.*

I burst into tears and couldn't stop crying.

I knew then that one of the reasons Gary had arranged for me to come to the Outback was so that he could say good-bye and convince me to move on. It was his way of saying, *Hey kid, I'm passing the torch to you. Time for you to live your life fully, and continue the work. You're doing such a great job. I am so very, very proud of you.*

I had tested myself and passed. I had faced the rigors of the Outback—the heat, the cold, the insects, the uncertainty—and I had stayed upbeat and available. I had stepped up to help the other women in their emotional work. I was respected and people believed that the words from my mouth contained what they needed—that they came from Divine Love. I had worked with the Aboriginal women in their important spiritual work and contributed power to the ceremonies. I had begun to realize my own power—the power that Gary knew I had all along.

Here in Australia and in the Outback, I had come to know what I had to offer, just as Gary had found his own healing powers here those many years ago. I was no longer Gary's adjunct. I had begun to see what my purpose was in remaining here on Earth without him. I had important work to do.

It felt like a rebirth in the womb of the planet, Uluru.

I had to hurry and board the waiting truck with the other eight women crammed into the back. Although all the other women in the truck were exclaiming over the sight of Uluru in its rare rain-soaked purple glory, my eyes were too filled with tears to see it.

56

THE RIGHT ALIGNMENT

When I returned from the Outback, it was made very clear to me that I needed to leave the house I had shared with Gary. What Gary had told me on my final walk in the desert had struck home. It was time to move on. An even more amazing life awaited me, and I had been empowered enough by my experiences in Australia to embrace it.

I had put the house on the market more than a year ago, but it had not sold. Given that I was still holding on to it in my heart, that wasn't surprising. After my experience in the Outback, I expected the team would immediately provide a buyer, but that is not what happened. I was astonished to find the house still didn't immediately sell.

Eventually, I invited Karyn to come in and check the energy. "Wow," she said upon entering the house. "Gary's energy is still so strong here. No wonder it's not selling." I had thought I let go, but I was so comfortable with all our shared belongings in the house that it never occurred to me they were creating a deterring energetic block to someone else seeing the place as their new home.

I packed up a number of Gary's things and moved them to a storage locker. Still, despite the zealous marketing of my realtor, there wasn't even a nibble.

How I wish I could say that, after my empowering experiences in the Outback, I waited patiently for the house to sell, knowing it was all being taken care of by my awesome spiritual team.

Sadly, I cannot claim that.

Even though I had discovered my own spiritual potency and even though I had added Auntie Ella and a number of other wonderful Aborigines to my spiritual team, I railed and complained. My Checker-helping mind danced and rampaged all through the selling period, wreaking havoc on my peace of mind. Once we've done our part by providing the "what" (what we want to have happen), it is so hard to give up the "how" and the "when." All my busy, worrying mind accomplished was to make me thoroughly miserable during the wait.

But Divine Love was working its plan as usual, delivering perfection to everybody involved. My newfound inner confidence eventually won out. I learned valuable lessons during that period: that there are no idle thoughts, the importance of concentrating only on what I wanted and not on what I didn't want, what tools were best for me to use to focus, and how to use self-love to encourage myself to let go of outcome and achieve peace. The frustrating time during which my house did not sell was a laboratory for my newfound inner power and a chance to equip my spiritual tool belt.

Late in the fall, Lynn stopped by with lunch. Ever the sweetheart, she wanted to cheer me up and make sure I was doing well. As we were munching on bean burritos at the kitchen table, the phone rang. I swallowed and picked it up.

"Hello." I listened intently to the person on the other end. Then, "You're kidding!" I practically screamed into the phone.

Lynn swiveled around in unbridled curiosity. She was kept hanging because it was a one-sided conversation. I was listening in silence with my mouth open in delighted shock.

Finally, it finished up. "Of course! Yes, I'll be here. Thank you, Beth. Thank you!" I hung up the phone and threw my arms in the air.

Lynn stood up from the table and started walking toward me. "Tell me! What's going on?"

"You won't believe this. Oh my gosh, I've got to sit down." I slowly made my way over to the kitchen table and sat. It was such a relief after all this time, more than a year. I felt as light as a helium balloon.

Lynn sat back down at the table and patiently waited. (She always was the patient one in our family.)

"My realtor, Beth, says we've a bidding war on our hands," I said, still breathless.

"A bidding war, what do you mean?"

"Beth says there are two different buyers bidding on my house at this very moment. She's coming over right now with both offers." I clapped my hands and bounced in my chair like a kid.

"After all this time, out of nowhere you've got two different people who both want to buy this house on the same day?"

"Can you believe it?!"

"I wonder who the buyers are," Lynn mused.

"Beth said one of them is Randy, the contractor who fixed the bedroom ceiling when the tree fell through," I told her. "I wonder why it took him so long to decide to buy it."

"I know he admired the solid construction when he was repairing the bedroom, and he told me several times how much he loved the view," added Lynn. "Who would have thought a tree going through the roof would bring in a buyer just when you needed one."

"I knew he had something to contribute. Randy's a helluva nice guy. He bent over backward for Gary and me. I'd love to see him in this house. Knowing the new owner will love it as much as we did will make it so much easier to hand it over. I'm going to do my best to make sure he gets it."

"And you thought the team wasn't taking care of you," Lynn chided me.

"Yeah, I knew better. I just got scared." I suddenly felt compassion for the heartbroken widow I had been. I knew my team wouldn't want me to blame and beat myself up for being only human.

Within twenty-four hours the offer was signed.

Randy would soon be the new owner.

My next task was to find a place to live.

Since my trip to the Outback, it had become much easier for me to leave the home Gary and I had shared. I could feel he was with me no matter where I went, so I knew I could move to any area I wanted. Where should I be looking?

I had developed some easy ways to get messages from my guides: I could use the pendulum; I could muscle test by asking my questions and letting my body give me a yes or no answer; I could ask the question and wait for synchronistic messages through friends, written material, or even signs and billboards. I now had so many ways to receive guidance from them. This time I was told very clearly that I would find a place in Richards, the town where my sister had found her apartment. Of course! That would be perfect. I settled down to wait for Gary and my guides to help arrange it.

Again there was a delay. I had to move out of the Keyserville house and into two separate rental houses before Divine Love created the proper alignment. But this time—I'm happy to say—I had the tools to endure the wait with grace. I kept checking in with my team daily. I kept practicing my meditation and taking good care of myself. I stayed focused on the perfect place. It was a done deal. I would be in it as soon as Divine Love decided the time was right. There was no doubt.

One day, I was preparing some dinner when the phone rang.

"Hello."

"You gotta get over here right away!" Lynn shouted over the line.

"You okay? What's going on?"

"I just saw my neighbor putting a 'For Rent' sign on the house right next door to me. It's the cutest little house. Get over here before somebody nabs it!" Lynn was frantic.

"I'll be right there." I put down the spatula and turned off the stove.

I left the dinner half cooked, grabbed my jacket, and started down the road.

It was rush hour and traffic was heavy. My heart seemed like it was beating out of my chest. My intuition told me this place was to be mine. It just felt right, even though I hadn't even talked to the owners or seen it. I kept repeating to myself, "If it's supposed to happen, it will. If it's supposed to happen, it will."

Waiting at a red light a few miles from Lynn's apartment, I glanced out the window and saw a popular Internet provider's truck. Written over the entire side of the truck in huge red letters was "Clear Channel."

"Cute," I said out loud. "I've got the funniest team."

I pulled up next door to Lynn's apartment where there was a "For Rent" sign hanging on a wooden post in the front yard. Lynn was eagerly waiting on the sidewalk out front. I barely got out of my car when Lynn ran over. "Look at how sweet the yard is. I know it's tiny, but I think it's darling."

I looked at the cozy white house with blue trim. I looked at the flower-filled yard. The back door was about forty feet from Lynn's carriage-house apartment. "I love it," I said, putting my hands on my heart, unconsciously repeating the gesture Lynn had made when she first saw her apartment.

"I never park in the front, but today I forgot my yoga mat and parked here to run in and get it. When I came back out, the guy was just putting up the sign. I just happened to glance over and see him. Don't you love the synchronicities?!"

I was afraid to get too excited. Part of me didn't want to go through the anguish of losing out on this great house right next door to my sister. It would be a more perfect arrangement than I had dared to hope for.

"What a kick to live next door to each other!" Lynn was beyond excited, but the *yeah-buts* arising in my mind were starting to drown her out.

"Lynn, this beautiful house in this beautiful neighborhood—everybody's going to want it. There will be a list of potential renters as long as the block in twenty-four hours. I can't see them picking me over the others who'll want to live here." I hated hearing the negativity in my voice.

"I think it's supposed to happen. There are too many synchronicities," Lynn declared.

Just then a car alarm across the street went off for no apparent reason.

We looked at the empty car, then at each other, and both burst out laughing.

57

HOME IS WHERE . . .

Three months later I was pulling weeds in my backyard and listening to dozens of birds chattering away in the tall evergreens, talking all about their day with great enthusiasm. I stood up to stretch my back and glanced around my cozy yard filled with flowers.

After the move next door to Lynn, my life had settled into simpler routines at a slower pace, and my mind and body thrived on it. The house was a tiny cottage and I was surprised at the emotional freedom that came from having fewer possessions. With fewer things to take care of, my life was so much simpler. Gary would be pleased to see me—gasp—often slowing down, quieting my mind, sitting on my back patio sipping tea.

I yanked a dandelion out of the soft ground, which was tender from the recent rain. Suddenly a hummingbird buzzed close to my face then flew into a nearby rhododendron. He and I were old friends, but recently the tiny bird had become protective of the area around the tall, thick bush. I moved away suspecting the shrub now held a nest with eggs. *Don't worry. I'll give you some space, little guy.*

I decided to take a break and plopped into one of my patio chairs. The sun was warm and I pulled off my garden gloves one by one and laid them on the glass-topped table. I breathed in the scent of some nearby jasmine and turned my face up to the summer sun. I should be taking advantage of the good weather to finish my weeding, but I let it go.

So many good things had come into my life recently, and I had found it was all about letting go and making room.

It took another year after my Outback trip, but I finally became ready to open my life to romantic love again. I looked around my house, around my bedroom. I had pictures of Gary, mementos of Gary, and gifts from Gary everywhere. I was sleeping under the beautiful spread that had been on our bed. Slowly, lovingly, I gathered up the pictures, the wind chimes, the altar, the love mementos, the possessions of his that had reminded me of Gary every day and moved them to my office. Gary was still very present in my work. This was a good room to be reminded of Gary. I would meet him there to continue our inspiring work together.

I stripped the spread off the bed and bought a new one.

Within a week, someone new had come into my life. It felt comfortable. It felt fun. We laughed a lot.

I knew unequivocally Gary had been waiting for me to be ready to do this—he had wanted this for me. Having a boyfriend didn't mean I needed to deny my ongoing relationship with Gary. It just meant I needed to get very clear that the romantic part of our relationship had ended. It was what Gary wanted, what he had encouraged me to do in the Outback desert walking the sacred Aboriginal grounds. He was waiting for me to let go and be happy in love again.

It didn't mean I loved Gary any less. He still always had fresh flowers by his picture and a red rose on our special days. He was still in my heart. Hearts are elastic that way. My heart was big enough to hold all the love.

All the love. There hasn't been a moment I wasn't surrounded by it. It was Saturday and my sister was coming over later with a spinach lasagna for our weekly dinner with a card game and a movie. But judging by the position of the sun in the afternoon sky, that wouldn't be for a while. This warm Saturday afternoon was the perfect time for a little reflection on life.

Everything was expanding for me. I was finishing Gary's book and I was set to publish it. I was publishing articles and reaching out through web pages on the Internet. I had found the perfect set of people to support and help me with those tasks. My speaking and my counseling were going well. I was traveling across the country and even around the world, speaking and sharing. The messages that Auntie Ella had told me to spread were being enthusiastically embraced wherever I sent them, wherever I went.

How on Earth had I gotten here? I found myself so in touch with Divine Love, feeling so cared for. I certainly hadn't always felt this way. It seemed like I had weathered some incredibly hard struggles and felt very alone at times. Yet the rocky roads I had traveled had been my personal route to ending up here. What could I subtract and still have gotten to this point?

I knew the Aborigines taught Gary that everything happens for a reason. The Aborigines believed everything that comes to us is to be richly experienced, learned from, and then released with gratitude. You acknowledge the gifts and then you move on to the next experience.

Gary had been grateful in the end for his MS. Could I find gratitude for the illnesses that nearly killed me? The Aborigines had advised Gary to let go of his abuse story. That it was actually a gift. Could I let go of my victim story: how I almost died from a blood transfusion tainted with hepatitis C, how the experimental treatment put me through hell and almost killed me?

What was the gift in those almost fatal circumstances? I took a deep breath and tried to see it from the perspective of my life now.

Well . . . being so sick for so long gave my family and friends the chance to care for me and show how much they loved me. I also learned I was stronger than I knew and that I had to take responsibility for my health. I learned I could be my own hero. And I learned the only way for me to heal was to make the choice to take better care of myself and love myself back to health. Now there was a lesson with lifelong benefits.

It seemed like the deeper I delved the more gifts I came up with. There were more gifts to surviving and healing the hepatitis than I had realized. Surviving such slim odds woke me up and put me on a quest to find Divine Love. Wow. I had to think about that for a minute. The best gift from the hepatitis was discovering the Divine is within me. And that the Divine is in everyone and everything around me. That was a huge gift! Really, it was *the* gift.

I sighed deeply, breathing in the realization that what started with a tainted blood transfusion had brought enormous blessing into my life.

A little voice inside me wanted to raise a question. *How about being a widow, losing my dearest love?* I could feel my throat tighten and anger start to well up in my chest. *Where the hell was the gift in losing Gary?*

Instantly, I heard in my mind, *Sweetheart, I'm always here with you. Now I can help you and others more than I could in a physical body. You've done such a great job of letting me go.* The warmth that I felt when I heard Gary in my mind released the tension and the anger. It seemed to dissipate in an instant.

That's true, sweetie, I spoke to him in my mind. *You've shown me plenty of signs that you're with me. I know you're helping me. Thank you, love.*

Reflecting on it for a moment, I realized I'd grown stronger since Gary had passed. I was finding my own power. Moving on to the next adventure, whatever it might be—and it was shaping up to be pretty spectacular. Gary, Divine Mother, and the Aborigines had taught me well. They had taught me how to heal, how to release my mind's controlling grip, and how to let them help me. Now I might be able to help others do the same.

My next thought made me smile. *The hardest things in my life have been my strongest teachers.* Each one has been one of my greatest blessings.

I could feel a beautiful calm ripple through my body. That beautiful glowing warm energy seemed to flow through me and out and around me. I felt a strong peace in my heart, an inner glow, and it was remarkably soothing—I was giving myself the peaches and cream treatment!

With a big smile spreading across my face, I whispered, "It's been a long journey but I remember now. It feels good to be home."

58

PARIS

I was once again traveling—this time in France. It was 2010, and through another series of coincidences, synchronicities, and miraculous financing, I had been invited to join a group of amazing women who were traveling around France following the trail of devotion to Mary Magdalene. There were twelve of us.

We traveled all over the south of France, and everywhere we went I had it in the back of my mind that Gary and I had planned to visit this very area when he could walk. At each field and vineyard, each picturesque town, I wondered if I was walking some of the same land Gary and I had walked together before in other lives.

The others in the group quickly learned that where I go, Gary goes, and they welcomed him. One of the women on the journey was Natasha, a lovely Australian woman with huge eyes and long, flowing black hair. She was having some knee trouble. We had been walking all day, over many days, over sidewalks, cobbles, up hillsides, even over rough fields. Unbeknown to me, she asked Gary for some help healing. She did experience a healing. The pain was gone and she was able to walk again over the rest of the trip without trouble.

Natasha expressed her gratitude to Gary profusely in her mind and asked him if there was anything she could do to thank him. Evidently, he gave her explicit instructions.

Some time later, I was standing in the kitchen of our rented French farmhouse and Natasha approached me, a little shyly. "Robbie, I hope you don't mind that I have been interacting with your husband who has passed. I don't mean to be meddling in your affairs."

"Not at all," I assured her. She was holding her hands behind her back and I couldn't guess what was coming.

"Well, you know I asked Gary to help me with my knee and that now it's better."

"That's good," I said.

"Afterward, I asked him, 'Is there anything I can do for you to express my gratitude for this experience?' And I got an answer. As clear as day. One sentence."

"Gary was always very succinct."

Natasha then drew a red rose from behind her back and handed it to me. "He said, 'Give Robbie a red rose for me.'" The rose was wrapped in cellophane, tied up with a red ribbon. Natasha was going on about how surprisingly difficult it had been to find one, but I'm afraid I wasn't listening. I was gazing at my rose.

It was one of those timeless moments when eternity hangs in the air. Natasha could not possibly have known how much that simple gesture meant to me here in the south of France.

Our last stop was Paris. The hotel room was tiny. The people were not rude. They were respectful and even friendly, just as Gary said they would be.

The Seine, the river that Gary and I had always dreamed of walking along, looked a little drab that day. The flowers he had talked about weren't out yet, and it was cold and rainy. But I didn't care. As I walked the lower path that runs right along the bank, I knew a deep peace.

Gary was with me the whole time.

He is with me now and always.

We may not be walking hand in hand, but we are certainly walking heart in heart.

CONTINUING THE JOURNEY

We invite you to continue your experience. Visit our website at **www .holzwellness.com** where you can:

- Read about Gary and Robbie's award-winning book *Secrets of Aboriginal Healing: A Physicist's Journey with a Remote Australian Tribe*
- Learn more about the remote Australian Outback Aborigines
- Read Robbie's blog, including how to work with your spirit guides and angels
- Buy Robbie's online course and integrate the Aboriginal healing steps into your life
- Learn about Robbie's forthcoming books
- Schedule a consultation with Robbie on how to create the life you love
- Discover more tips on utilizing the power of your mind and help from a Greater Consciousness
- Purchase Robbie's guided meditations and other body/mind/spirit wellness products
- Invite Robbie to speak to your organization
- Buy additional copies of *Aboriginal Secrets of Awakening* and *Secrets of Aboriginal Healing*

We'd love to hear from you. Contact us at **info@holzwellness.com**.